Chaos, Creativity, Completion

Chaos, Creativity, Completion

New Approaches to Writing and ADHD

EDITED BY CHLOE MARTINEZ AND
LISA VAN ORMAN HADLEY

Foreword by Rebecca Makkai

The University of Chicago Press   Chicago and London

The University of Chicago Press, Chicago 60637
The University of Chicago Press, Ltd., London

Published 2026
Printed in the United States of America

35 34 33 32 31 30 29 28 27 26 1 2 3 4 5

ISBN-13: 978-0-226-83493-1 (cloth)
ISBN-13: 978-0-226-83495-5 (paper)
ISBN-13: 978-0-226-83494-8 (ebook)
DOI: https://doi.org/10.7208/chicago/9780226834948.001.0001

Library of Congress Cataloging-in-Publication Data

Names: Martinez, Chloe editor | Hadley, Lisa van Orman, 1979– editor | Makkai, Rebecca writer of preface
Title: Chaos, creativity, completion : new approaches to writing and ADHD / edited by Chloe Martinez and Lisa Van Orman Hadley ; foreword by Rebecca Makkai.
Description: Chicago : The University of Chicago Press, 2026. | Includes bibliographical references.
Identifiers: LCCN 2025032523 | ISBN 9780226834931 cloth | ISBN 9780226834955 paperback | ISBN 9780226834948 ebook
Subjects: LCSH: Attention-deficit hyperactivity disorder | Creative ability—Psychological aspects | Creative writing—Psychological aspects
Classification: LCC RC394.A85 C43 2026
LC record available at https://lccn.loc.gov/2025032523

♾ This paper meets the requirements of ANSI/NISO Z39.48-1992 (Permanence of Paper).

Authorized Representative for EU General Product Safety Regulation (GPSR) queries: **Easy Access System Europe**—Mustamäe tee 50, 10621 Tallinn, Estonia, gpsr.requests@easproject.com
Any other queries: https://press.uchicago.edu/press/contact.html

A Note on the Type

This book was designed with both neurotypical and neurodivergent readers in mind. The text is set in Neue Haas Unica, a sans-serif typeface chosen for its clean, uncluttered shapes and friendly feel. The text is left aligned to keep spacing between letters and words consistent, and to allow for flexible line lengths—both of which can help make reading easier.

Contents

Foreword

REBECCA MAKKAI

In sixth grade I showed up for school one day wearing pink corduroys and a sweatshirt covered in neon swirls. This medium-cool look was fairly standard for me in 1989, as were my messy hair and dirty sneakers. I was, as usual, running late.

What wasn't usual: stares and confusion from the rest of the class, someone asking, "Why are you wearing *that*?" Everyone else, I realized, was wearing extremely formal clothing for a Tuesday morning. Coats and ties, dark dresses, polished black shoes. I sat with them on the floor (this was a Montessori school and, thank god, I was never stuck at a desk), and someone reminded me that we were attending the funeral of our classmate's father that day.

"Reminded" is a strange word here, because I had absolutely no idea that this was happening. I was very aware of this man's passing, and I might have known (I can't remember now) that there was going to be a service at some point. A permission slip may have been involved. But the fact that we were piling into parents' minivans and heading to a church was absolutely news to me. I don't mean that I went "Oh shoot, that was *today*?" I mean if I walked into your home right now and asked if you were ready for your space mission—that's how unexpected this was.

I was incensed, really, that no one had told me. I hadn't missed school recently, so the announcement must have been made when I was in the bathroom. I believed this for years, until I looked back and recognized that the incident fit a much larger pattern of missing details, zoning out, being essentially absent even when my body was right there. This remains true even today. In a group listening situation—say, when a fellow author is giving a reading—it's like I'm listening to a radio station that won't quite come in. Sometimes I get a sentence or two, and then it's gone. Then a word, then fuzz. Telling myself to focus does as much good as telling myself to listen harder to a broken radio.

We went to the service, and I felt as self-conscious as an eleven-year-old girl can, which is *very*. I was also aware enough to realize that this wasn't about me, and that the real problem was showing disrespect in a tragic situation. My negligence was actually offensive this time.

Throughout that year and the surrounding ones, my garden-variety preteen awkwardness was compounded not only by a sense that I couldn't do anything right but also by a teacher who felt the need to point this out in front of everyone. I was clearly lazy—or else why couldn't I get assignments done despite testing through the roof on aptitude? I was messy, always losing things, my papers always crumpled, my handwriting a mess. I couldn't organize my time, especially without a pressing deadline. I was forgetful. I was clumsy and uncoordinated, on top of which I couldn't focus on anything athletic for more than a few seconds at a time. (I got through ballet class by pretending that we were being filmed for an antiperspirant commercial. I kept this up for at least a year.) I was impatient, unable to make myself take the time to screw lids back on paint or to use a ruler. I fidgeted constantly, but not in ways most people would notice; I folded and refolded my tongue, or I moved my toes in a pattern. In a nifty OCD-ADHD crossover, I amused myself in any moving car with windshield wipers on by imagining laser beams coming out the end of each wiper and making sure the beams lined up both with the trees we were passing and the white stripes on the road. Mostly, I was "spacey." I could (and still can) uphold my end of a simple, otherwise logical conversation by going "Okay, right . . . sure . . . got it," when I had absolutely zero idea what was being said or what I was agreeing to. My mother would tell me when and where she'd pick me up, and then ask me to repeat it back to her. Usually I couldn't. Teachers would wave their hands in front of my face and say, "Earth to Rebecca," in some approximation of an alien robot voice. This was considered, in the '80s, an absolutely hilarious thing for teachers to do to students.

At no point during this time—in fact, never in my life—did anyone suggest that I might have ADHD. Of course, diagnoses were relatively rare then and tended to be reserved (and still tend to be reserved) for the kids causing actual disruptions in class. Those tended to be boys. More specifically, they tended to be white boys: white boys who couldn't sit still, who blurted out interruptions, who threw things or drew on the table or ripped a math page to shreds in frustration. If a child of color did those things, it was typically considered a discipline problem, not something neurological. And the vacant stares of girls like me weren't disruptive, so we just got scolded for our late or missing work and were mostly left alone again to doodle listlessly in our notebooks. We weren't nominated for special testing, because why would you test for what was so clearly laziness?

A lot of people with childhood ADHD allegedly "grow out of" the condition. I don't quite understand how you can grow out of having a certain kind of brain, though, and I suspect we're often mistaking coping mechanisms for a change in chemical makeup. What I do know is that anecdotally there's a huge number of adults working in the arts or other creative fields who have ADHD, and there are a whole lot of women who only get diagnosed when their children do (and when they finally see a list of symptoms written out). I owe my own diagnosis not only to such a list but also to other adult women with ADHD speaking frankly about how their minds function. Several years ago I read an essay by the author Robin Black about her ADHD, and I marveled that someone like that could possibly write books. *How awful that must be for her!* I thought. *How strange!* The writer Kim Brooks, a close friend, told me about her ADHD, and while I still didn't see myself reflected, I did notice that we both worked a *lot* better under pressure. Then I heard the writer and podcaster Sarah Marshall, whose brain seemed to work much like mine—highly associative, full of metaphors—refer frequently to her ADHD, and something small clicked into place.

I started writing about ADHD in my Substack newsletter in 2023, and the response from other women, particularly other women writers, was overwhelming. Within a month, seven of them had gotten officially diagnosed, and ten more told me they were in the process of pursuing a diagnosis. Quite a few people also commented that while they didn't have ADHD, they related to every single thing I'd described. (I think they're still picturing the stereotypical ADHD poster child, that little white boy throwing spitballs.)

I'm on a mission now to not only describe my own experiences (which you might or might not see yourself reflected in) but also talk about the unsung strengths that often come with the condition. Because I *love* the way my brain works. And I want my sixteen-year-old, who also has ADHD, to love the way she thinks as well.

First of all: It's busy in there. I take it there are some people whose brains are like quiet country roads, focused on one thing at a time. My brain is like Times Square on a Friday night. And not the picturesque Times Square on a postcard, but the chaotic parts where people run around in Elmo costumes. At any given moment, I have at least one song in my head, plus other words that are not the words I'm actually thinking or the words of the song. Both those words and the words I'm thinking or saying or hearing, I picture all of them spelled out. Every letter has a color, and every word has a color that's usually—but not always—an average of those colors. I'm also keeping track of rhythms and patterns I'm making with my tongue and my toes and, depending on the situation, laser-beam windshield wipers. And I'm thinking of several other things that are not part of the topic at hand—memories and possibilities and the fact that I looked up Matthew Broderick this morning on Wikipedia and then ended up on his father's Wikipedia page and learned that he was in a Broadway show called *Johnny No-Trump* that closed on opening night, and that I want to go back and look up more about this play later and try to figure out if the Mary Mercier who wrote it is the same Mary Mercier who was married to Gene Wilder and had a small role you'd probably remember in the movie *Airplane!*

But ADHD also comes with periods of intense hyperfocus. My daughter hasn't cleaned her room in weeks (because it's boring and annoying), but right now, as I write this, she's been cleaning and organizing for ten hours straight. I offered to watch TV with her for a break, and she wasn't interested. She's in the zone.

You know what two things you really need in order to make great art? A mind that teems with possibility and association and creative detail but which can also focus—intensely, for long periods of time—on creative obsessions.

There are certainly people who make art but don't have ADHD, and there are certainly people with ADHD who don't make art and are fine with that. I don't know any of the latter, actually, but that's probably because most of the people I know who aren't artists are humanities professors who need the exact same skill set. In other words: Everyone I happen to know with ADHD is in exactly the right career. There might be neurodivergent accountants out there—and maybe they've found a way to happily maximize their skills—but I wouldn't have had the occasion to meet them.

To be clear, ADHD is a disability. It interferes with my daily life in unpleasant ways, and even now that I know why I am the way I am, I'm still furious with myself daily for some oversight or failure to finish work or lack of organization. My inability to schedule doctors' appointments or refill prescriptions on time is downright dangerous. But these frustrations are more about clashing with a world not built for me than with disliking my own mind.

It's not fair, but someone put the morning people in charge of the world, and *they're* the ones making the workday start at 9:00 a.m. Someone put the country-road-minded people in charge of lower education, and they're the ones making students focus on one subject at a time and stare straight ahead at a chalkboard and grading them on whether they use a ruler. (A Montessori education helped me, that one critical teacher notwithstanding, by being an amorphous hole for my weirdly shaped peg. I could spend an entire week writing a play, and then catch up on math the next week. I wish everyone had that option.) Someone went and invented clocks and calendars and email and decided that clothes shouldn't be wrinkled. Someone invented paperwork and decided that getting a mammogram should involve fifteen online forms and three different logins.

As the world recognizes more and more neurodivergences—and accepts them as vital, not as sad accidents of nature—we can surely find a way to make the world more *ours*. The contributors to this anthology are doing that, if only by writing about a reality that a reader might relate to strongly or might have never even imagined. One of the traps of being human (or more specifically, a singular human person) is that we assume, until confronted with the evidence, that everyone else's brain works just like ours. For the neurotypical, this means absolute confusion about why other people aren't able to make things work easily, why they can't just motivate themselves to get organized and focus and get things done. For the undiagnosed neurodivergent, it means you tell yourself that *everyone* has racing thoughts constantly, *everyone* finds it easier to write a novel than to put clothes away, *everyone* starts ten projects and finishes none of them, *everyone* "struggles with attention sometimes" (by which everyone else means they can get momentarily distracted, and *we* mean we've been walking around in a thick brain fog our entire lives). We think that surely *everyone* is so curious about the world that each word or moment or thought is like a hyperlink you might follow into infinite, rhizomatic pathways of information and ideas. It's quite sad that for some people, that last one isn't the case. What a disadvantage! Let's call their condition Attention Simplicity Disorder. Let's try to tolerate them in school when they write down uncreative, single-minded answers and don't even doodle in the margins.

(I need you to know that apparently Bernadette Peters made her Broadway debut in *Johnny No-Trump*. I just spent ten minutes on her Wikipedia page instead of writing this essay. This led me to the page for *The Horn and Hardart Children's Hour*, for which Fred Rogers worked as a stage manager. Apparently, he and Tom Hanks are sixth cousins. Tom's father was "an itinerant cook," which sounds fascinating, but the trail ends there.)

What you're about to read are the windows into fifteen writers' worlds and minds, ones we're all lucky to find ourselves invited into. Because what's better than a kinetic brain? What's better than someone who's endlessly open to the world and its infinite possibilities?

Welcome to Times Square. I'm the one in the Elmo suit, handing you a flyer to an experimental all-night show in the basement of a condemned restaurant. You're going to love it.

Introduction: We Saved You a Seat (Sitting Is Optional)

LISA VAN ORMAN HADLEY AND
CHLOE MARTINEZ

A couple of years ago, the two of us sat at a table facing a sea of writers—our colleagues—in a large convention center ballroom, feeling a mix of excitement and terror. We were about to reveal a secret that we had spent much of our professional lives trying to cover up: We have ADHD. We worried that our audience would think we were scattered, hyper, undisciplined. But we were also sick of nodding along to traditional writing advice that just didn't seem to work for us. We were ready to crack the door open on our writing lives and talk about how ADHD poses unique challenges for us but is also the source of extraordinary gifts.

We began our panel by encouraging the attendees to fidget, draw, ask questions—whatever would make them feel comfortable and tuned in during our conversation. As we talked with the other panelists about how ADHD informed our writing, we laughed and cried together and, yes, we lost track of time. And everyone else—the other writers in the room—they got it, got *us*. They *were* us. People rushed up afterward to show us their knitting projects and handmade pencil cases. They told us that they were buzzing with ideas for their own writing projects. They asked whether we had any additional resources we could share with them on writing and ADHD. Aside from a few online articles, we couldn't find anything to suggest to them. But then we remembered: We have always had to find new tools, new pathways. The book we were looking for didn't exist yet, so we decided to create it ourselves.

*

What might be one of the first descriptions of ADHD is found as far back as the fifth century BCE, when Hippocrates described a type of "soul," or intelligence, that "rapidly passes judgment on the things presented to it, and on account of its speed rushes on to too many objects." He believed these characteristics indicated an imbalance of the "humors" (too much fire! not enough water!), and prescribed hydration and exercise, moderation in sex and alcohol, and eating a good meal before work, "as their soul is more stable when it is mixed with its appropriate nourishment than when it lacks nourishment."[1] Not the worst advice, really.

Fast-forward about two millennia to an eighteenth-century German medical textbook called *Der Philosophische Arzt*. The author, Melchior Adam Weikard, devotes an entire chapter to attention deficits within a larger section titled "Sicknesses of the Spirit." He describes, somewhat poetically, a person with such a "sickness": "Every humming fly, every shadow, every sound, the memory of old stories will draw him off his task to other imaginations. Even his imagination, if and when it is copious, entertains him with a thousand minor subjects." Weikard cites poor upbringing as the cause. His recommended course of treatment includes cold baths, dark rooms, horseback riding, sour water, and silence.[2]

1 Hippocrates's *Regimen* 1:35, cited in *Handbook of Neuroscience for the Behavioral Sciences*, vol. 2, ed. Gary G. Berntson and John T. Cacioppo (John Wiley & Sons, 2009), 1020; for a translation of the full text, see Hippocrates, Volume IV, Heracleitus, *On the Universe*, trans. W. H. S. Jones (Harvard University Press, 1931), 289–91.

2 Russell A. Barkley and Helmut Peters, "The Earliest Reference to ADHD in the Medical Literature? Melchior Adam Weikard's Description in 1775 of 'Attention Deficit'

Since the publication of that German textbook, there have been many different (and, frankly, kind of rude) names for this condition, including "abnormal defect of moral control," "clumsy child syndrome," and "minimal brain damage." In 1968 a diagnosis called "hyperkinetic reaction of childhood" first appeared in the *Diagnostic and Statistical Manual of Mental Disorders* (*DSM*). In 1980 the name of the diagnosis was changed to Attention Deficit Disorder (ADD) with and without hyperactivity, and in 1987 it was changed again to Attention-Deficit/Hyperactivity Disorder (ADHD). In 1994 ADHD was further broken down into the three presentations—predominantly inattentive, predominantly hyperactive/impulsive, and combined—that we use today.[3] Our understanding of the source of ADHD has also evolved. It is now understood not as an imbalance of fire over water or a case of bad upbringing, but a neurodevelopmental condition with a strong hereditary component.[4]

Despite this long history, in many ways our cultural and medical understanding of ADHD is still in its infancy. Until the 1990s, ADHD was associated mainly with hyperactivity in boys, and even in recent decades, it has been underdiagnosed in girls and in adults, not to mention in people of color.[5] However, intersectional understandings of neurodiversity are beginning to become more widespread, alongside a major cultural shift toward acceptance and acknowledgment of disability and difference. We now seem to be in a unique moment of "unmasking" around neurodivergence, disability, and mental

---

(Mangel der Aufmerksamkeit, Attentio Volubilis)," *Journal of Attention Disorders* 16, no. 8 (2012): 623–30, https://journals.sagepub.com/doi/10.1177/1087054711432309.

3 Jeffery N. Epstein and Richard E. A. Loren, "Changes in the Definition of ADHD in DSM-5: Subtle but Important," *Neuropsychiatry* 3, no. 5 (2013): 455–58, https://pmc.ncbi.nlm.nih.gov/articles/PMC3955126/.

4 Stephen V. Faraone and Henrik Larsson, "Genetics of Attention Deficit Hyperactivity Disorder," *Molecular Psychiatry* 24, no. 4 (2019): 562–75, https://pmc.ncbi.nlm.nih.gov/articles/PMC6477889/.

5 Noha Shalaby, Sourav Sengupta, and Jamal B. Williams, "Large-Scale Analysis Reveals Racial Disparities in the Prevalence of ADHD and Conduct Disorders," *Scientific Reports* 14 (2024), https://www.nature.com/articles/s41598-024-75954-5.

health—of beginning to own and share our differences in social, educational, and professional spaces rather than working to camouflage and compensate for them. Even the increasing popularity of the nonmedical term "neurodivergence" acknowledges a shift in our understanding, a turn toward treating brain differences as unique traits rather than disorders. The number of people diagnosed with ADHD is large and growing[6] and, given findings that people with ADHD are particularly adept at tasks related to creative cognition,[7] the incidence of ADHD among writers is likely to be even higher than in the general population. This book gathers the wisdom of a few of those ADHD writers.

*

When we began to think about how we would approach this project, we read up on anthology editing. The advice seemed to say: "Don't even attempt to edit a collection of essays unless you are an extremely organized person. You must be detail-oriented. You must be able to stick to an editing schedule and find contributors who are able to meet firm deadlines." It may as well have said, "Ask a doctor whether you and your contributors have ADHD before proceeding. The risks associated with putting together an essay collection if you have ADHD include rejection, humiliation, and failure."

When we told others about the project, the response was often something along the lines of "Wow—so you're soliciting new essays and prompts from *thirteen* writers with ADHD?! That sounds like herding cats!" Our response: "Well, we really like cats. We, too, are cats."

6 That number is now estimated at more than fifteen million in the United States. Brooke S. Staley et al., "Attention-Deficit/Hyperactivity Disorder Diagnosis, Treatment, and Telehealth Use in Adults—National Center for Health Statistics Rapid Surveys System," *MMWR Weekly Report* 73 (2024): 890–95, https://www.cdc.gov/mmwr/volumes/73/wr/mm7340a1.htm.

7 Holly White, "The Creativity of ADHD," *Scientific American* 30, no. 3 (2019), https://www.scientificamerican.com/article/the-creativity-of-adhd/.

And yes, we encountered some challenges along the way. We took alternate routes that were overly complicated but also scenic. We were excited to figure out the best way to stay organized, so Chloe made a Trello board that we both stopped using after a few weeks, and Lisa made a color-coded tracking spreadsheet that only Chloe ended up using. We made a Jamboard that we only used once. We made Google Docs and then we made copies of those Google Docs and copies of *those* Google Docs. We got confused about which version was the most up-to-date.

We missed some deadlines, and our authors did too. We underestimated the amount of time it would take us to comment on all of the essay drafts—because what even is time? But when we sheepishly wrote an email telling the contributors that we were running a little behind schedule, they wrote back with so much support and validation. "No problem at all," they said. "We get it!" We set ambitious goals for ourselves that we could not always meet. We got sidetracked in research wormholes. We spent too long double-checking that the email we were sending included the correct attachment. We struggled to keep track of our process, maybe because we changed that process each time we discovered that it was no longer working.

And all that was *fine*. In fact, it was perfect.

What we already knew from our own writing lives was true in this case as well: neurotypical tools and practices don't always work, particularly for a book about neurodivergence edited by two neurodivergent people. In creating a collection that imagines new possibilities for how to write with ADHD, we were also able to imagine new possibilities for how to edit an anthology with ADHD. But unlike the solitary experience of working on our own books, this time we had each other.

We discovered, working together virtually from Utah and California, that collaboration was the ADHD hack we had been looking for. It allowed us to motivate each other and problem solve, hand difficult tasks back and forth, and provide each other with structure and accountability as we balanced this project with our already-hectic work and family lives. We experienced, for the first time, what it was like to work with someone in our own neurotype: to be able to tell each other that we couldn't get anything done for six hours, then got a huge thing done in the fifteen minutes before school pickup; to talk over one another sometimes and use too many exclamation points in emails; to ask each other when we needed help. Seeing ourselves in each other helped us get past our shame about how we work, and also helped us see the value in our unique approaches.

Once, Chloe printed something out and cut it into pieces so she could rearrange them on her office floor, and when she sent a picture of these scraps of paper to Lisa, Lisa immediately replied with a picture of her own floor covered in cut-up pieces of the same piece of writing. Lisa started a lot of things that Chloe finished, and Chloe was enabled to do a lot of things because Lisa had taken the first step. We had long Zoom coworking sessions. In the final stages of the project, we retreated to a tiny red house on a working farm in Utah and spent a few intense days writing and editing, with breaks to hike and eat and swim in a geothermal pool. We were "body doubling"—using each other's physical presence as motivation to stay focused through the challenging homestretch.

We report all this not just to tell you what a great time we had, but because it feels important: In making this book, we were able to work in ways that worked for us, with others who were like us. In the small community of ourselves, our own (wonderful!) editor, and our contributors, we considered for the first time what we really needed, and how we could do our best work. It made all the difference. Getting to read the essays in this collection was a huge part of that difference. We learned from our contributors and saw ourselves in their brilliant essays, finding shared experiences but also seeing new ways of writing that we had never considered. As each new essay rolled in, our belief in why this collection was so important grew. It wasn't just a book that other people needed. It was a book that we ourselves needed. The process of putting it together taught us that two people with ADHD *can* edit an essay collection.

And why was anyone ever trying to herd cats in the first place? We aren't herd animals.

Until now, many ADHD writers have been left to figure it out on their own. This book aims to lessen that burden by offering hard-won wisdom, inspiration, and techniques from accomplished writers from many genres and professions. These writers share—with openness and enthusiasm—their personal experiences, some of the strategies that have helped them, and the unexpected ways that ADHD shapes their work. They also show, in their approaches to the essays, how terrifically creative ADHD writers can be, writing in experimental forms (see Douglas Kearney's kaleidoscopic visual piece), engaging beyond the page (like Khadijah Queen's piece, with its stage directions drawing our attention to a real person in a room speaking), and embracing simultaneity and sidetracks (see Jennifer Knox's wildly inventive essay). Other essays intermingle research and personal experience (Teresa Dzieglewicz), poetry and prose (lawrence-minh bùi davis), and stream-of-consciousness description (Allison Adelle Hedge Coke), just to name a few.

These essays consider how we might write in ways that embrace rather than mask our neuro-difference; tell stories of diagnoses that have come, in many cases, as midlife revelations; and offer multiple ways of finding writing practices that work for us—practices that often look quite different from traditional writing advice.

Many of our contributors have also included a writing prompt after their essays. We hope this will make for a more interactive reading experience. We also hope these prompts will spark new ideas, help you generate fresh work, offer ways of revising that you might not have tried yet, or allow you to discover new writing practices that work for you.

We wanted the book to include the perspective of someone with professional training related to ADHD. We are writers, after all, not doctors or therapists or neuroscientists. The closing chapter features a conversation with David Kessler, a licensed therapist and nationally recognized ADHD advocate.

We've included a glossary of terms that have been helpful for us in understanding what is going on in our brains and making sense of our lived experiences. Some of these come from neuroscience and psychology while others are nonscientific terms used in neurodivergent communities.

Finally, we have included a list of recommended resources, from books and websites to our favorite timers and gadgets. Since language, the internet, and the ADHD community are constantly evolving, these can only ever be a snapshot of the moment from which we write; nevertheless, we hope they're of use.

A note on terminology: We have chosen to use the current official diagnostic term Attention-Deficit/Hyperactivity Disorder (ADHD) throughout this book.[8] While we like that this term unites us rather than dividing us based on specific symptoms,[9] we also know that "ADHD" can't fully capture the range of our experiences. For example, it doesn't acknowledge things like hyperfocus, emotional regulation, time agnosia, creativity, and struggles with executive function—all things that many ADHD folks experience. We also take issue with the language of "deficit" and "disorder." We hope a different name will take its place in the future—one that acknowledges the complexity of this neurotype and that captures its positive aspects in addition to its challenges.

When people first asked us to point them toward resources on writing and ADHD, we didn't have much to offer them. But now we do. With this book we are enthusiastically flinging the door open on our ADHD

8 *Diagnostic and Statistical Manual of Mental Disorders: DSM-5*, 5th ed. (American Psychiatric Association, 2013).

9 Some people still use "ADD" and "ADHD" as separate terms to denote the lack or presence of hyperactivity.

writing lives. We hope these essays and writing prompts will make you feel a little less alone in your writing practice, and a little more like you are sitting in a room full of like-minded people in eccentric outfits who *get* it. We saved you a seat—no matter who you are or what diagnoses you have (or don't have)—but feel free to get out of your chair, interrupt, doodle, knit, bounce your knee, play with your necklace, take breaks, and let your mind wander during our conversation. We hope you will feel validated in your particular experience of writing and your way of navigating the world. We hope you will feel proud of everything you figured out on your own before you got here: all the spectacularly creative solutions you came up with, perhaps without even knowing you were doing so. And we hope you will feel emboldened to fling the door of your own writing life wide open. Welcome. It's an extraordinary space. You're right on time.

1

Lisa Is a Joy to Work With. She Does Not Know What Happened to Her Health Project.

LISA VAN ORMAN HADLEY

When I was eight, my dad had me take the Myers-Briggs personality test. There was one question on it that completely baffled me: "Is it worse to be in a rut or have your head in the clouds?" When I told him that I didn't understand the question, my dad explained that "being in a rut" means you're stuck doing the same things over and over, and "having your head in the clouds" means you're daydreaming and disconnected from reality. "Yes, yes," I said, "but the part I don't understand is why someone wouldn't want to have their head in the clouds? It's wonderful."

I had two recurring dreams as a kid. The first was that I was a mermaid businesswoman. The second was that I lived in the clouds. I couldn't fly, but I could bounce around from cloud to cloud and cover huge aerial distances that way. I was the most expansive version of myself up there.

*

A couple of years ago, my mother handed me a gallon-size Ziploc bag with my first name written in Sharpie across the plastic. Inside, I found a stack of pink progress reports, from kindergarten to sixth grade. I wondered what they would say about me.

I remember being a shy, daydreamy kid with a desk crammed full of papers. Each time I added a new one, all the other papers had to bend themselves into new shapes to make room for it. I identified with those papers, identified with constantly contorting myself to fit into spaces that didn't seem made for me, though I could never quite figure out why.

I learned best through reading and doing, but my brain would switch off as soon as the teacher stood at the front of the classroom and started talking. Well, that's not exactly true. My brain does not have an off switch—it just changes channels. My teacher, probably noticing that I had tuned into an inner broadcast, often called on me suddenly. Sometimes I caught just enough of the question to guess at an answer, but other times I was left to explain myself. Why hadn't I been listening? Did I need to be sent to the school nurse to have my hearing checked?

I started reading the reports aloud to my mother:

Kindergarten: *Lisa likes to do things in her own way and in her own time.*

First grade: *When Lisa settles down, she can do "A" work. She needs to learn to concentrate on the right things at the right time.*

Second grade: *Lisa is a joy to work with. She does not know what happened to her health project.*

Third grade: *Lisa needs to work on assuming responsibility for her work, glasses, etc. I'm proud of Lisa's "A" in reading. She has a lot of potential.*

Fourth grade: *Writes original, excellent compositions.*

Fifth grade: *She works very hard.*

Sixth grade: *Lisa is a bright student. Her listening skills and socializing during class are her weaknesses. Lisa's report on Clara Barton is well-researched. She still needs to turn in her note cards and bio cards.*

Two things were clear to me by the time I finished: (1) I was a writer, and (2) I had ADHD.

I stuffed the papers back into their plastic bag, threw my hands into the air, and shouted, “How in the world did we miss my ADHD for so many years?”

*

We missed it for forty-two years to be exact.

We missed it because, when I was growing up, no one was thinking about a brain like mine existing in a body like mine.[1] Back then, if we thought about ADHD at all, we thought of little boys ricocheting off schoolroom walls and hallways like pinballs, setting off lights and sounds and endless bonus rounds. It didn’t even occur to us that girls could have it.[2] If ADHD boys were like pinballs, ADHD girls were like game pieces that had been knocked to the floor and lost under the couch. We were stuck there for decades among the stretched-out bobby pins and crusty pennies and eddies of cat hair, not knowing what game we belonged to or whether we even belonged to one at all. Some of us are still there.

By the time I entered middle school, no one—especially me—could understand how I could score above the 99th percentile on the California Achievement Test yet have a column of D’s on my report card punctuated by a single A in English. One morning in eighth grade, I walked into my life science class to find that all the desks had been pushed together to form a half circle. My teacher, Mr. Browning, had come up with a “brilliant experiment” the night before: Our seating assignments for the remainder of the year, he said, would be based on our performance in the class. He then pointed to the first desk and announced the name and grade of the top student. The kid with the next-highest grade was told to sit at the second desk.

1 The first meta-analysis on gender differences in ADHD wasn’t published until 1997, the year I graduated from high school. M. Gaub and C. L. Carlson, “Gender Differences in ADHD: A Meta-Analysis and Critical Review,” *Journal of American Academy of Child and Adolescent Psychiatry* 36 (August 1997): 1036–45, https://doi.org/10.1097/00004583-199708000-00011.

2 Not to mention transgender and gender-diverse individuals.

Mr. Browning continued around the half circle, calling out lower and lower grades, until there was one name left. I took the last seat and tried to play it off like I didn't care.

Of course I cared. The message that I was a failure wormed its way into my core, oxidizing everything it touched. I don't know what conclusions Mr. Browning landed on after analyzing the data from his experiment, but *my* takeaway was that I was a bad apple. It has been estimated that by age ten, children with ADHD have already received twenty thousand corrective or negative messages from their teachers.[3] Using the progress reports I got from the outside world as a blueprint, I started writing my own progress reports and handing them out to myself. I was lazy (even though I never stopped to rest). I was dumb (in all the ways that actually mattered). I had my head in the clouds (and that was the wrong place for it).

I didn't know how to change who I was, so I found a few friends to help me fit in. Their names were Masking, Perfectionism, Hypervigilance, and occasionally Class Clown. They *did* help at first. But then those friends started bringing *their* friends over, uninvited. Unlike my hand-selected companions, these guests were wild and destructive. Their names were Self-Loathing, Social Anxiety, Overwhelm, Treatment-Resistant Depression, Disordered Eating,[4] and Intrusive Thoughts. They devoured my confidence, got me in trouble, and left behind a whole lot of messes.

3 Michael S. Jellinek, "Don't Let ADHD Crush Children's Self-Esteem," *Clinical Psychiatry News*, May 1, 2010, 12, https://www.mdedge.com/psychiatry/article/23971/pediatrics/dont-let-adhd-crush-childrens-self-esteem.

4 While this might seem unrelated, a 2007 study by Harvard Medical School found that adolescent girls with ADHD are almost four times more likely to develop an eating disorder than their non-ADHD peers. Joseph Biederman et al., "Are Girls with ADHD at Risk for Eating Disorders? Results from a Controlled, Five-Year Prospective Study," *Journal of Developmental and Behavioral Pediatrics* 28, no. 4 (August 2007): 302–7.

A few weeks before my mother handed me those progress reports, a psychiatrist had finally, after more than four decades, handed me a diagnosis. There was the immediate grief of wishing I'd known sooner, of wondering how my life could have been different if I had understood this about myself. ADHD felt like a decades-long secret my body had kept from me. It made so much sense in retrospect, but I couldn't understand how all the disparate parts of my personality fit together until I was given this specific map—until I saw how the rivers of forgetfulness connected to the forked pathways of attention, how the mountains of impulsivity dropped off into deep canyons of rejection sensitivity.

My new diagnosis explained so many things I had assumed were personality quirks at best and moral failings at worst. It explained why I wanted to jump out of the car every time we passed a certain gas station and my twins yelled out, "Mom, remember that time you drove away with the gas pump still attached?" It explained why I couldn't sit still, why my therapist said our sessions felt like a game of Whac-A-Mole, why I swung wildly between not being able to focus and not being able to stop, why I dove headfirst into new hobbies only to abandon them as soon as they didn't feel new anymore, why I walked into a room to perform one task and ended up doing one-tenth of ten other things instead.

But once the fluorescent shout of all my ADHD-induced failures dimmed to a whisper, I heard another voice, a voice I hadn't listened to in a long time. My inner broadcast was gently asking: *What if nothing was wrong with you in the first place? What if the real problem is that you paid too much attention to all the progress reports from the outside world saying that your way of doing things is wrong? What if the clouds were a soft place to land all along?*

It was a quiet, seismic shift. It changed everything.

Okay, not everything. I'm still constantly second-guessing myself. I'm still terrified of failing, of people seeing me fail. Sometimes I wonder whether I became a writer and editor because I am so practiced in editing myself. Right now, for example, I am worried that you, my reader, are thinking, *What does any of this have to do with writing?* I have rewritten this essay so many times, and each time I've tried to get to the writing part sooner. But every time, I keep coming back to the progress reports, all the negative messages I've taken in. They're at the root of most of my struggles with writing. They're at the root of most of my struggles, period.

Ernest Hemingway famously said in an interview, "The most essential gift for a good writer is a built-in, shockproof, shit detector."[5] He said this at the end of a kind-of-hard-to-follow rant about Graham Greene and gaggles of geese and yearbook editing (god, did *he* have ADHD too?), so while I'm not completely sure of what he meant by it, this is what it means to me: Along with all the messages I've received about who I should be as a person, I've internalized a lot of messages about who I should be as a writer, from when and how I should work to what a story should look like. Have you ever been told that a writer should sit in a chair for *x* number of minutes every day, that they should write *y* number of words, that the best time to write is *z*? If so, I invite you to throw that out because it's bullshit. A writer is a person who writes, full stop. What and when and how you write is up to you. The ADHD writer's first task is to be a shit detector. We must identify and root out all the ableist lies we have been handed before we can learn to trust the cadence of our own minds and the power of our own voices.

I am acutely aware of all my failures. But instead of constant self-editing, I'm ready to point my red pen outward, to examine the messages I received and edit the shit out of them.

It's time to do some shit-detecting in my progress reports.

5 Ernest Hemingway, "The Art of Fiction No. 21," interview by George Plimpton, *Paris Review* 18 (Spring 1958).

“When Lisa settles down, she can do ‘A’ work”

At the beginning of my MFA program, my supervisor looked over the stories I submitted as part of my application and told me I was doing it wrong. She said that my stories should be at least ten pages long, move linearly through time, and be invented (“It’s hard to believe this is fiction when all your characters are named Lisa, Lisa”). I felt immediate shame, as if I had been caught cheating on a test. And then I panicked. I had never written the kind of story my supervisor was asking for. I didn’t even like *reading* those kinds of stories. I had applied to the fiction program because I didn’t know where I or my writing fit in. I was drawn to experimental stories that lived in the liminal spaces between worlds, stories that snipped at the imaginary threads separating fiction from autobiography, comedy from tragedy, poem from prose. But I did not have the confidence back then to challenge the messages I got from those in positions of authority. Instead, I bought into the idea that my way was wrong.

I was expected to submit new work every three weeks. I would spend the first week filled with so much anxiety about what to write that I couldn’t write anything. Then I would spend the second week hating myself so much for not having written anything the first week that I still couldn’t write anything. Near the end of the third week, full of self-loathing and fear of disappointing my supervisor and classmates, I would force out a ten-page story featuring lackluster characters who marched in a straight line toward their denouements. Those stories bored the hell out of me and made me feel like I was walking in a straight line toward my own denouement as a writer.

I was matched with a new supervisor for my second semester. He was gossipy and kind and a little irreverent, which immediately put me at ease. He must have sensed that I was spinning out in a literary rut, that I had lost my voice and my motivation. He encouraged me to play around on the page without worrying about what I was making and whether it was okay to make that.

When I was a kid, my brothers and I loved to play around with text. We used BIC pens to cross out words on our cereal boxes and create erasure poems from the words that remained. We carefully cut out pieces of the headlines from last week's newspaper and spliced them together with the current week's headlines, then eagerly watched as our dad opened the paper in front of his bowl of raisin bran and started to read our absurd, dark creations. My brother Jonny, an artist, could perfectly mimic our dad's handwriting. One day Jonny found a message our dad had written to our older sister on a notepad next to the telephone: "Amy, Erika called at 5:13 p.m. Love, Dad." Below the signature, Jonny added in our dad's handwriting, "Also, you are a nerd." Amy's distress over our dad calling her a nerd sent us into fits of laughter for weeks. It was that playfulness—the power of words to delight and surprise and reinvent—that first made me fall in love with writing.

So I returned to the familiar tools of my childhood. I wrote a Choose Your Own Adventure about discovering that my grandmother wore a wig. I replaced words in the poem "There was an old woman who lived in a shoe" with blank, underlined spaces to create a Mad Libs–inspired poem about women's lib. I wrote one-sentence stories whose entire livelihoods depended on their titles; a list of reasons why no one signed up for my mother's sewing class; a six-act play about puberty; and a glossary of the peculiar phrases my parents used.

During his 2018 commencement speech at the Columbia Journalism School, Ira Glass said, "It's traditional in this sort of speech to give advice. I will not do that. Except this: amuse yourself. . . . Everything will be better if you're out for your own pleasure."[6]

Not all stories are meant to amuse, of course. I was writing about hard things—my dad's Alzheimer's, my four failed rounds of IVF, the

6 Ira Glass, "Ira Glass's Commencement Speech at the Columbia Journalism School Graduation," *This American Life*, May 17, 2018, https://www.thisamericanlife.org/about/announcements/ira-glass-commencement-speech.

murder of a family friend. Since I was writing about my family, there was also the question of how they would react. But the *way* I was writing amused and energized me. It motivated me to keep pushing through all the narrative knots and hard feelings.

Settling down was bullshit. Settling down drained the life out of my stories. I was only capable of "A" work when I got up and played around.

"The right things at the right time"

Here is a strange thing about me: I frequently confuse the words "yesterday" and "tomorrow." I cannot seem to place the right things at the right time. So I am constantly saying things like "Tomorrow I took the twins to the park" and "Yesterday I will organize my closet." (Google Docs underlined the wrongness of those verb tenses in red as I wrote them; it probably also knows that I will never *actually* organize my closet.) I used to say this problem with chronology was because I am omnipresent, but now I wonder whether it's just another aspect of my ADHD: time agnosia, or a slippery relationship with time and how it passes.

There was one story that I couldn't find a way into. When I was seven, my neighbor from across the street was murdered on the side of my house in the middle of the night while knocking on our windows and begging for help. She was a friend of my mother's and the first person I knew who died. The story was literally and emotionally so close to home that I had a hard time seeing it clearly. I had a kind of story farsightedness and no matter which lens I tried, I couldn't seem to correct it. Then, as one last Hail Mary, I tried flipping the narrative upside down and telling it in reverse. When I did that, all of the ribs of the story suddenly slid into place.

Much later, I did an exercise in the book *Drawing on the Right Side of the Brain* that helped me understand why reverse chronology helped me break through the hard exterior of that story. The exercise was called "Upside-Down Drawing: An Exercise That Reduces

Mental Conflict."[7] It asked me to reproduce an upside-down copy of Picasso's *Portrait of Igor Stravinsky*. Since the image was rotated 180 degrees, the hands didn't look like hands, the eyeglasses didn't look like eyeglasses, and the pocket square didn't look like a pocket square. Instead, I saw lines and the spaces between them. As I began to draw, I didn't feel mentally conflicted at all. I had one simple task: to make lines that branched out to other lines. When I was done, I flipped my drawing right-side up. I was amazed to see that it was not terrible. In fact, it was the best copy I had ever managed.

Similarly, flipping my story upside down removed my expectations of what I was looking at. It removed my farsightedness, creating the distance I needed to see the events, people, and emotions objectively. It helped me focus on how each story line branched out to other story lines: the evolution of our friendship with the neighbors, the life cycle of the cicadas in our Florida neighborhood, the comings and goings of our cats, the murder. It allowed me to see connections I wasn't able to see when looking at the story head-on.

Reverse chronology also just *felt right*. The part of my brain that mixes up yesterday and tomorrow finally had its moment in the sun. Its weird talent for putting the wrong things at the wrong time saved the story. I titled it "Irreversible Things," which would eventually become the title of my book.

"Lisa needs to learn to concentrate"

People often ask me how I came up with the idea to write that book the way I did—the unusual way it moves through time, the unconventional containers, the blurring of genres. Before my ADHD diagnosis, I didn't know how to respond to those questions. It just kind of *happened*, I said. But now I have an answer: I wrote my book the way I did

7 Betty Edwards, *Drawing on the Right Side of the Brain*, 4th ed. (Tarcher, 2012).

because I have ADHD. My book wasn't a departure. It was coming home to the way I think.

My brain doesn't work chronologically. It doesn't tell me stories about my life in a linear way with predictable pacing. It doesn't know how to draw a line between memory and fiction or how to untangle one emotion from another. It's a wild animal. It runs on instinct and impulse. It capriciously follows scent trails and stops to lick itself mid-hunt. I try to feed it and keep it comfortable: I use noise-canceling headphones to block out ~~my kids and spouse~~ distractions,[8] knit sweaters to calm my anxiety and rage, practice planning ahead and problem-solving while rock climbing twice a week, take my meds, go to therapy. But I've found that one of the best things I can do for my attention is to let it take *me* for a walk.

When I let my brain off leash and follow its associative meanderings, it shows me delightful things I never would have found otherwise. My feral brain gnaws on obsessions and narrative knots, turning complex ideas that seemed impenetrable into something soft and workable. It tracks emotional weight, sensing the right moment to pounce. It gathers disparate images and weaves them into a nest that holds. Sometimes it takes a good, long nap. My untethered attention notices things in the tall grasses that it couldn't have seen if it had remained on the marked path. And it always manages to find its way home.

I didn't need to learn how to concentrate; I just needed to embrace how *I* concentrate.

"Weak listening skills"

The biggest obstacle to writing for me isn't time, even though my twins and freelance work keep me pretty busy. It isn't a lack of dis-

8 I am sad to report that I have since broken these very expensive headphones by repeatedly falling asleep on top of them.

cipline or passion or tools or talent (but I would like more of each, please). It isn't laziness, although I used to mistake it for that. No, the thing that knocks me out of my writing chair again and again is listening too well, allowing messages from the outside to dull my ability to hear myself. It is tuning into frequencies that say I am not good enough, that my way of navigating the world is flawed. In kindergarten, my teacher said I liked to do things in my *own way* and in my *own time*. But by first grade, suddenly there were *right things* I wasn't doing and a *right time* in which I wasn't doing them. I wish I had never perceived that shift. I wish I had listened less to all those messages and instead turned inward, homing in on the natural inclinations of that little kid with her head in the clouds who did things "in her own way and in her own time." That kid knew her own expanses.

My kindergarten progress report reminds me of the Maori word for autism, *takiwatanga*, meaning "her own time and space." Not a disorder; a unique way of experiencing the world. The Maori word for ADHD is *aroreretini*, meaning "attention goes to many things." Not a deficit; a bounty.

I am working on writing a new progress report to myself: *Lisa thinks outside the box because she can see now that there is no box. There was never a box. The people who think there is a box are confined to narrow spaces, stuck in a rut. Instead of a box, there are clouds, and it's more than fine—wonderful, in fact—to spend time in them.*

After editing the shit out of my progress reports, I was able to see the helpful messages that were there all along. My teachers said I was bright and I worked very hard. They said I wrote original, excellent compositions. They said I was a joy to work with. They said I had *potential*, a word I always used to interpret as "you're not good enough." But come to find out, that word has always meant *power*.

PROMPT: I See a Head in the Clouds

When I was a kid, one of my favorite activities on cross-country road trips was to have my brothers make a random squiggle on a blank piece of paper. I would then use my pen to transform the squiggle into, say, a picture of a long-nosed dog in a party hat riding a slightly skewampus unicycle. The starting squiggle took away my anxiety about where and how to begin. Like looking for shapes in the clouds, it allowed me to see images and stories that I wasn't able to see when staring up at the blank sky. This prompt is meant to remove the feeling of overwhelm at the thought of making something from nothing by repurposing things that have already been written.

- Find a note someone has written to you (or a progress report!) and alter the narrative by crossing things out, adding footnotes, and/or giving it a title.
- Take a preexisting short story, essay, or poem—your own or someone else's—and alter the narrative by flipping it upside down and telling it in reverse or reshuffling the contents. See what new connections emerge when you remove the expectation of a predictable chronology.
- Cut two headlines out of a newspaper and assemble the words or groups of words into a new headline.
- Use a permanent marker to create an erasure poem on a piece of packaging from the recycling bin. Cross out words and let the words that remain tell a new story about the product or something else entirely.
- Alter a recipe you find online or in a cookbook by crossing out ingredients; suggesting substitutions; and/or adding a comment about how the recipe turned out, what it tasted like, and what memories it conjured for you.

2

Fruit from Space

Neuroscience for ADHD Poets

TERESA DZIEGLEWICZ

I've spent so much of my life feeling as if I had missed some prerequisite class for being a human. Like I'd been put to work in a rocket science lab without taking Physics 101. Or given a child's sketch of a house and asked to build a functional living space. But these gaping holes in my knowledge were instead around how to keep my room clean, how to shrink my emotions down to a normal size, how to build a bridge between my brain's wild leaps and the person on the other end of the conversation.

Ashamed of my inability to conform, I tried to live halfway undercover. Like an off-brand Dick Tracy, I attempted to wear normalcy like a big hat and trench coat. Writing was the one place where I could safely remove the disguise and let all the jagged pieces of myself spill out. Poetry was big enough to hold my brain's leaps, my *Hindenburg*-size emotions, my magpie obsession with small things and sensory memories. It was where I could be the most untranslated version of myself.

Perhaps I would have kept living this double life, but then I became a mother and learned that my wild radiance of a child is neurodivergent. At that time, ADHD diagnoses were also blooming like dandelions among my poet friends. It occurred to me that maybe this was not a coincidence, and the more I learned about ADHD, the more it resonated with my own experiences. I started to wonder: If I was trudging through the world wearing neurodivergence like a hair shirt, what kind of message would I be sending my child? How could I teach someone else to love their ADHD brain when I spent so much time hating and hiding my own? I began to consider, too, how the pieces of me that I had been so busy covering up had perhaps also gifted me the refuge I found in writing.

Since I've been diagnosed with/discovered my own ADHD, I've kept thinking about these questions. Could understanding the connection between ADHD and poetry be a foothold, a stabilizing foundation on which I might begin to make peace with my neurology? I recently recruited a pair of knowledgeable and generous guides to help me find out: Dr. Holly White, a cognitive psychologist who researches ADHD and creativity, and Isabelle Richards, a therapist and cohost of the ADHD podcast *Something Shiny* (and also, to my great luck, my high school friend). White and Richards are not only experts on ADHD—they both also have it themselves. They were each kind enough to join me for some delightfully ADHD Zoom calls that included rescheduling, diversions about lamps and cauliflower rice, and me stimming so enthusiastically I got my pen stuck in my hair. The neuroscience I learned from these conversations deepened my understanding of my brain, allowing me to see its challenges and delights and strengths woven together.[1]

Wild Rivers of Attention

The "AD" in ADHD stands for "attention deficit." But my brain has never felt like an attention desert; rather, it overflows and sloshes with noticing. In fact, in our conversations, both Dr. White and Richards made the point that ADHD is more accurately described as an *abundance* or perhaps an *inconsistency* of attention. Dr. White analogized

1 All of the quotes and neurological explanations from Holly White and Isabelle Richards come from a series of interviews I conducted with them over Zoom in 2023.

ADHD attention to a rapidly swinging gate: sometimes flooding us with information, sometimes slamming closed. I began to picture my brain and attention not as an aqueduct but as a wild river of tributaries and estuaries, an overflow of sensation and emotion that isn't easily diverted or controlled.

The human brain's gray matter is a thicket of nerve fibers and ricocheting neurons that allow our brain to talk to itself. For people with ADHD, the gray matter that connects our prefrontal cortex with our sensory centers and amygdala is weaker than average.[2] This means that the bossy, grown-up prefrontal cortex has less control over the more free-range feeler and thinker inside us (the amygdala)—in other words, it has less ability to snap its efficient fingers and say *pay attention*.

While this cognitive mismatch can make some things very challenging (in my case: taxes, not leaving my phone in the fridge, a general belief in "time"), it can also create a heightened sensory experience. Dr. White explained that once the gate of attention swings open, ADHD brains literally cannot stop noticing. When I move through the world, I'm often distracted by a tree root shaped like a curled-up cat, the call of a bird I don't recognize, the backfire of a car, or a song playing down the street. I interrupt conversations to say, "Did you see that? Did you hear that?"

Emily Dickinson wrote, "If I read a book [and] it makes my whole body so cold no fire can ever warm me, I know that is poetry."[3] We feel poems not only in our minds but also in our bodies. And those swarms of details winging through the gates of the ADHD brain? When crafted into a poem, they can create a richer and more embodied experience for our readers. Recent research on mirror neurons

2 Martin J. Batty et al., "Cortical Gray Matter in Attention-Deficit/Hyperactivity Disorder: A Structural Magnetic Resonance Imaging Study," *Journal of the American Academy of Child and Adolescent Psychiatry* 49, no. 3 (2010): 229–38, https://pmc.ncbi.nlm.nih.gov/articles/PMC2829134/.

3 Emily Dickinson, letter to T. W. Higginson, August 16, 1870, https://archive.emilydickinson.org/correspondence/higginson/jnl342.html.

suggests that reading a sensory detail can actually activate the corresponding sensory center in the brain.[4] So if I write the words "the sound of a fork scraping against a plate," your brain might light up as if you yourself have actually heard that metallic screech. When you read the Dickinson line, did you feel the cold within your skin?

This wild noticing also creates transcendence in art. Ross Gay's poem "To the Mulberry Tree" begins with the should-be-disgusting moment of a bird pooping in the speaker's mouth.[5] However, the speaker, through an intensive noticing of the sun on his chin, the bird in a branch above, even the precise texture and flavor of, yes, the shit itself, transforms this experience from something base to something near sacred. Poetry's bright scattershot of focus can contain the tools of transformation.

And that rampant ADHD amygdala, (relatively) unconstrained by the prefrontal cortex, guess what else she controls? *FEELINGS*. And if there's anything I know, it's that poets love a feeling! While a neurotypical person may be able to compartmentalize their feelings, regulating emotions can be more difficult for those of us with ADHD. Neuroscientist Dr. Joel Nigg (who decidedly does not appreciate the gifts of the ADHD mind, and whose work I do not otherwise recommend) has said that people with ADHD experience "a lot of emotional suffering because they're being buffeted hither and yon by their emotions."[6] And, yes—I *am* buffeted hither and occasionally yon. When asked about my writing process, I often joke that the first step is to "journal and cry" (spoiler: this is not actually a joke). Both Dr. White and Richards compare emotional dysregulation to a lack of "brakes." I'm strangely tickled to imagine my neuroses and enthusiasms as a rickety bicycle careening downhill.

4 J. M. Kilner and R. N. Lemon, "What We Know Currently About Mirror Neurons," *Current Biology* 23, no. 23 (December 2, 2013), https://doi.org/10.1016/j.cub.2013.10.051.

5 Ross Gay, *Catalog of Unabashed Gratitude* (University of Pittsburgh Press, 2015), 74.

6 Joel Nigg, "'You're So Emotional!' Why ADHD Brains Wrestle with Emotional Regulation," ADDitude podcast, April 19, 2023, https://www.additudemag.com/webinar/emotional-regulation-adhd-anger-management-podcast-316/.

Richards also pointed out that not only are those with ADHD less able to control their feelings, but a craving for stimulation often means that their brains *desire* those big feelings (even difficult ones) in order to activate neurotransmitter chemicals like dopamine and norepinephrine. This form of self-medicating can create giant full-bodied feelings of joy, for which I am grateful. As many an ADHD person (and my therapist) can attest, it can also be very unpleasant. But perhaps it allows us to sit in the bigness of being human in a way that might be challenging for some neurotypical people. In his essay "A New Way of Living," Jericho Brown writes that the poem is singular in its ability to cause an emotional reaction in readers, and that "this change of mind leads to a change in action (or to changing inaction)."[7] It follows, then, that the world may need some people who can feel in ways that are not always convenient, and that it is this very disruption that may lead to meaning and change.

Ideas from Space

"Inhibitory control," or the ability to manage our own impulses, also impacts our ideas. According to Dr. White, in neurotypical brains, inhibition can come along and clip the strangest buds of thought off the vine before the thinker even registers them. This helps a person focus and prioritize. However, the ADHD brain tends to be a little more lenient with those pruning shears. While following a single line of thought might come in handy while filling out insurance forms, art often benefits from an ability to break with convention. In one experiment, Dr. White asked people to design a fruit from space (a fact that makes me want to start participating in cognitive psychology experiments).[8] Neurotypical people tended to design, like, a really

7 Jericho Brown, "A New Way of Living," Lambda Literary, April 3, 2018, https://lambdaliterary.org/2018/04/a-new-way-of-living/.

8 Holly White, "The Creativity of ADHD," *Scientific American*, March 5, 2019, https://www.scientificamerican.com/article/the-creativity-of-adhd/.

big banana. The fruit designed by those with ADHD was "more likely to include atypical features such as antenna, tongues, straws, and hammers." And if a space fruit unfurling its tongue is not a poem, then I don't know what is.

This lack of inhibitory control often leads to what Dr. White describes as an "accidental collision of ideas." I may be in a calculus lecture, but I'm thinking about the shoes of the person in front of me, the dinner I'm going to cook that night, the strange watermark on the ceiling (what could have made that?!). As a result, disparate subjects can become linked in my ADHD brain in surprising ways, which can often lead to more creative (and sometimes outrageous) outcomes.

Dr. White has studied this through word associations. She used a language analysis tool that measures the likelihood of finding two words together, and thus how much conceptual distance lies between them in the map of the brain. Her data shows that folks with ADHD tend to respond with words that are more surprising and less conventionally related. While explaining this to me, Dr. White delightfully interrupted herself to share how this phenomenon reminds her of an old Reese's Peanut Butter Cup commercial ("You got your peanut butter in my chocolate!" "You got your chocolate in my peanut butter!") and how the most innovative ideas often come from surprising blends. It turns out that mixing one's peanut butter into one's chocolate has a number of very useful applications in poetry!

In his book *Leaping Poetry*, Robert Bly describes an idea from ancient Chinese poetics that the poetic imagination is akin to "riding on dragons." He describes leaps from "the known part of the mind to the unknown and back again to the known," and he concludes that "the real joy of poetry is to experience this leaping inside a poem."[9] ADHD brains are literally wired to do this naturally: to move from one idea to the next in surprising ways.

9 Robert Bly, *Leaping Poetry: An Idea with Poems and Translations* (University of Pittsburgh Press, 2008).

According to Dr. White, this gift for cognitive leaping is also correlated with an ability to move quickly between the concrete and the abstract—in other words, seeing the connections between minute and grand details. Consider James Wright's "Lying in a Hammock at William Duffy's Farm in Pine Island, Minnesota," with its iconic ending, "A chicken hawk floats over, looking for home. / I have wasted my life."[10] Or Camille Dungy's "Trophic Cascade," in which she moves from a deeply detailed description of the gray wolf's reintroduction to Yellowstone to her own experience as a mother.[11] The impact of the lines comes from the surprise and quick oscillation.

It feels almost too obvious to mention that this associating of disparate things often kindles into metaphor. In one of my own poems, I describe the door handles of a car as swinging open like "the arms of startled infants."[12] This is a direct result of my attempt to write a poem while wondering if my child was successfully napping. Despite fervently wishing that I could focus on the poem, the metaphor only arrived because I was also thinking about the baby. My favorite metaphors in other people's poems also hinge on the unexpected—Ada Limón describing love as a newborn horse, or Sharon Olds comparing an erect penis to the eyestalks of a slug.[13] The word "metaphor" comes from the Greek word *metapherein*, meaning "to transfer." This process of transference, this overlaying of disparate ideas and objects and sensations, creates an experience that is entirely new, for both the reader and the writer. The caterwauling ADHD brain is built for this metamorphosis.

10 James Wright, "Lying in a Hammock at William Duffy's Farm in Pine Island, Minnesota," in *The Branch Will Not Break* (Wesleyan University Press, 1963), 16.

11 Camille T. Dungy, "Trophic Cascade," in *Trophic Cascade* (Wesleyan University Press, 2017), 16.

12 Teresa Dzieglewicz, "There Are No Police in This Poem," *Palette Poetry*, December 17, 2020, https://www.palettepoetry.com/2020/12/17/there-are-no-police-in-this-poem/.

13 Ada Limón, "What I Didn't Know Before," in *The Carrying* (Milkweed, 2018), 71; Sharon Olds, "The Connoisseuse of Slugs," in *The Dead and the Living* (Knopf, 1975), 51.

It's All About the Dopamine

As some of our parents might confirm, the ADHD brain can also be predisposed to risk and rule breaking.[14] The danger of a precarious ledge can be a real boon for those dopamine- and norepinephrine-hungry neuroreceptors. For the ADHD writer, poetry can provide this cliff—on emotional, intellectual, and craft levels. Contemporary poetry often involves making intimate emotions and experiences very public. (Sorry for the masturbation poem, Mom!) My very supportive husband, upon reading a particularly vulnerable poem of mine, has been known to remark, "I really believe in you doing this, and also I'm not sure why you want to."

During our conversations, Dr. White told me about a study she recently conducted on street artists. The study found that artists with nonlinear thought patterns were more likely to create multiple focal points; use unexpected colors together; leave shapes, lines, and images unfinished; and avoid drawing conclusions. This willingness to break with convention often resulted in stronger work (as measured, in this case, by a juried art show).[15] Similarly, the nonlinear propensities of many ADHD brains may support risk-taking on the page. Those risks not only satisfy our stimulation-driven neurology—they create art that lingers for the reader.

Even the idea of poetry as "the best words in the best order," as Coleridge famously said, might be attractive to the ADHD brain. When I told Richards how much I love hyperfocusing for hours, solving small puzzles of word choice and line breaks, she said this makes perfect sense. She explained that because ADHD brains "love some high stakes," the pressure and tension that poetry puts on each word, sound, comma, and line break could be giving me small hits of dopamine. Poetry doesn't require the explanations of prose—the struc-

14 "Other Concerns and Conditions with ADHD," Center for Disease Control and Prevention, https://www.cdc.gov/ncbddd/adhd/conditions.html.

15 At the time of the printing of this book, this study had not yet been published.

tured paragraph, the signposting, the clear evidence. It's a wilder bird, demanding perfection from each bone of its light skeleton in order to fly. In this way, our ADHD brains may not only contain the tools that help us craft the poems, but the poems may also contain the tools to ease our fluttering, hungry brains.

Rich Layers of Light

I want to be clear that just as those of us with ADHD shouldn't have to disguise our neurology in big hats and trench coats, we also shouldn't have to dress it in sequins for a talent show. Our value is inherent and doesn't come from something we perform or something we make. The science and conversations outlined here aren't meant to provide an argument that our ADHD brains are marketable. Instead, they have provided me with a new narrative for my neurodivergent brain, allowing me to see it not as a place of scarcity but of nuance.

When I view my life experiences and ADHD through the lens of poetry, they gain dimension and become holographic. Yes, there are many things that my brain is not built to do effortlessly. I will never be a person whose home is naturally spotless, who meets deadlines with ease, who doesn't leave my keys on the grocery store counter. But there are joys in this distractedness, in this untamed river. The porous banks let in surprise, let in rich layers of light. This is a story I can tell myself. This is a story I can tell my child. There is sustenance here and there is art.

PROMPTS: Weird Science

Color Prompt

Look around you, wherever you are. Choose one color that feels right to you. Give yourself fifteen minutes to freewrite about that color. What places does it remind you of? What memories? What sounds? What textures? Do some of these ideas, which may have otherwise seemed unrelated, mean something new once you put them together? Using your freewrite notes, write a poem. Use the color name as your title but don't mention it in the poem itself.

Word Association Prompt

Use a random word generator (like https://randomwordgenerator.com/) to generate a list of twenty words. Now look at each word on the list and write down another word beside it. This should be the first word that comes into your head; don't overthink it. Choose the five pairs of words that are the most surprising to you. Next, journal about an image or a memory that each word pair sparks for you. Finally, write a poem juxtaposing these fragments. What does it mean for these small stones of thought to live in a poem together? What other unexpected connections can you make?

Sensory Prompt

Divide a piece of paper in half. On one side, write "Sensory Details," and on the other side, write "Abstract Thoughts/Memories." Give yourself fifteen to twenty minutes to notice sounds, smells, textures, temperatures, ideas, anxieties, images, and more: both your external and your internal experiences. Jot down some notes about what you're experiencing on a sensory level on one side of the paper. On the other side, jot down some notes about the other thinking that's occurring in your brain. Write a poem that weaves some or all of these ideas together. If it feels right, try to avoid adding too many additional connecting words or ideas.

3

Writing into the *Wunderkammer*

DOUG VAN GUNDY

I don't know when I first saw the shadow boxes of artist and filmmaker Joseph Cornell. I may have been introduced to them through the poet Charles Simic's excellent monograph *Dime-Store Alchemy*, or I may have seen Cornell's shadow box *Untitled (Hotel Beau-Séjour)* in the Museum of Modern Art in New York when I was in my thirties. Even if you don't recognize Cornell's name, you've probably seen his work or the work of artists influenced by him. Cornell's meticulously constructed shadow boxes often contain collaged elements—illustrations, photographs, travel brochures, and other found and assembled objects—that half tell surrealist stories and then leave the meaning-making up to the viewer. His 1936 construction *Soap Bubble Set*, for example, contains clay smoking pipes, a porcelain doll head, a bird egg in a cordial glass, and a French map of the topography of the moon.

Cornell's packrat juxtaposition of images felt both surprising and oddly comforting to me. Looking at *Untitled (Hotel Beau-Séjour)* felt like looking into a mirror. Or rather, it felt like looking *through* a mirror, past the skin and bones of my face and into the shadow box of my own mind. The scraps of newsprint and advertisements in English and French that make up the back wall of the box are overlapping and incomplete, legible but fragmentary, like a transcript of distracted thought. Suspended in front of the text is a colorful paper cutout of a cockatoo, a showy, impressive bird capable of mimicking speech, but not of understanding the words it is saying. The metal pieces and cork ball—objects that are useful in other applications—are stripped of both context and purpose in the world of the shadow box. As a person with fragmented thoughts, a profound case of impostor syndrome, and the frequent feeling that I am useless at the tasks I attempt, *Untitled (Hotel Beau-Séjour)* was a visual text that felt like it was made for me. Recognizing these parts of myself in Cornell's work allowed me to consider the possibility that the way my brain works might be useful—especially in making art or poetry—instead of broken and shameful.

*

I have always been drawn to collections—dioramas in natural history museums, display cases full of mineral specimens, junk shops and antiquarian bookstores, my own childhood shoebox museums filled with pebbles and marbles and shells and matchbooks from diners and the stubs of pencils too short to sharpen. At this very moment, I'm sitting at a desk littered with pens, pencils, binder clips, erasers, glue sticks, highlighters, wood screws, three lighters, metal polish, violin rosin, a label maker, a fragment of an English porcelain saucer, an egg timer, a bicycle headlamp, and a glow-in-the-dark Super Ball painted to look like a human eye.

I realized early on that my collections and clutter drove my mother crazy. Many kids resist cleaning up after themselves but eventually learn to do so. Not me. As a child, I "cleaned" my room using the "object impermanence" method: if I couldn't see it, it wasn't there. I put everything that was on the floor—my clothes, books, shoes, toys—into the huge wooden chest at the foot of my bed until it was too full to close. While cleaning out my desk on the last day of third grade, I found the homework I should have turned in on Halloween wadded up behind an overdue library book, the crayon-colored jack-o'-lanterns out of place in the June sunlight. In high school, I carried all my books in a backpack throughout the day because there was no room in my locker to store them between classes.

So long as the disaster was confined to my bedroom, my parents were relatively tolerant of my clutter. My teachers were less so. I don't think I ever had a teacher in my public school career who didn't suggest, at least once, that I was lazy or sloppy or slovenly or a Venn diagram encompassing all three. Sometimes this was said overtly and at a high volume in front of my classmates. I found this particularly frustrating and demeaning because, try as I might, I couldn't do much about it in the long term. If I *really* focused, I could, painfully and with great effort, bring these external expressions of my internal condition into temporary order. But *temporary* is the key word. Before long, these spaces would fall back into the baseline state of chaos that simultaneously put me at ease and underlined my shame. Again and again I tried, and failed, to put the chaos behind me.

While my brain is obviously both the locus and engine of that chaos, I've never thought of my mind as "cluttered." The way my brain works makes perfect sense to me—after all, the inside of my skull is my normal and my thoughts are my mother tongue. I was in my twenties before I realized I was constantly translating from the language of my thinking into the language everyone else seemed to speak. This usually happened invisibly and in real time unless a distraction caused a lag in the process or I ran into some false cognate of cognition. Because of the organic and associative nature of my thinking, I frequently found myself seconds or minutes behind in conversation, as the natural flow of someone else's thought moved forward while I slowed down to explore the subtext, footnotes, and cultural history of whatever point the other person was making when I off-ramped back into my own thoughts. If my mother asked me to cut up an onion for the chili she was making, but then continued to a second point—asking if I wanted Fritos or cornbread with my soup—I was lost, already on some tangent that rendered me incapable of hearing what she was saying, much less acting on it—*Where are the botanical origins of the onion? France? It is* French *onion soup, after all. How do you say "onion" in French? Or "soup"? "Tureen" is a funny word; it makes me think of turtles. They do make turtle soup. What do turtles eat? Certainly not onions . . .* By the time I tuned back into what my mother was saying, she was frustrated and usually had moved on without my input.

I didn't just speak the dialect of reverie. I was also fluent in over-sharing, info-dumping, endless questioning, know-it-all-ism, and self-doubt. If I wasn't talking too much, I was disengaged from what was going on around me. If I wasn't trying to be the center of attention, I was trying to become invisible. If I didn't feel awkward and out of place, I was impatient as hell because people weren't talking or thinking fast enough. This informational, auditory, and emotional clutter followed me around like Pig-Pen's dust cloud. It was exhausting. It is still exhausting.

I eventually learned to mask my otherness and keep my enthusiasms to myself. I learned to look like I was paying attention in class so my mind would be free to wander and whir. I learned to pick up on incomplete information so I could pretend to care about sports or cars or hunting or whatever. After a while, this performative normality became second nature, a costume I put on before I left my bedroom in the morning and didn't remove until the end of the day. Only in creative work was I able to let my other self have free rein. When I was brainstorming, drawing, performing, and writing, my mind could finally stretch out to its full length like a dog who is finally let out after being penned up all day. When I engaged in these unstructured creative activities, I felt my mind leap and wiggle, run and bark, and *play*.

*

I finally received an ADHD diagnosis at age fifty-seven. While the diagnosis wasn't a surprise, the clarity and insight afforded by simply *having* a diagnosis was. I found one of my junior high school yearbooks recently. No fewer than *six* of the people who signed it used the word *weird* in describing me. *To a weird but good friend*, one read. *To a weird but cool guy*, read another. That *but* had the sting of a backhanded compliment. *Even though you don't fit in, you have* some *redeeming qualities*, it seemed to say. I could live with being weird, but I longed to be seen as weird *and cool*.

According to the online gallery Artchive, "Cornell's works are associated with Surrealism because of the unnatural assemblage of unrelated objects."[1] But nothing about these works feels unnatural or unrelated to me. Over the years, I've tried to share my enthusiasm for Cornell with others. A few already know about him or take a passing (or polite) interest. But some find Cornell, his obsessions and collections and constructions, *weird*. If pressed, they might say his shadow boxes are *weird but good* or *weird but cool*. I love these pieces precisely because they are weird. They ask questions that can't easily be answered. They put seemingly unrelated images and objects together so they talk to one another, and I feel compelled to try to understand that conversation. To me, Cornell's boxes are challenging *and* comforting—weird *and* cool.

Cornell's work asks to be viewed *associatively*. Just as a musical chord isn't located in any single note, but in how tones interact and interfere with one another, the arrangement of specific images in his shadow boxes creates meaning in the spaces between them. Sometimes, this meaning isn't particularly logical or easily translated into language and can only be understood on an emotional level. Whatever meaning you take from a Cornell box isn't inherent in the objects arranged inside; it is an emergent property of the arrangement as a whole. The mystery of this alchemy is what drew me to Cornell; it rewards the leaping way my mind works.

The opening poem in my first book, "Keeper," is in the voice of a brook trout who imagines what it would be like if he could breathe air instead of water.[2] My father is an aquatic biologist, and I spent a lot of time around rivers and streams as a child. In writing this poem,

1 "Joseph Cornell: Artwork and Bio of the American Sculptor," Artchive, April 6, 2023, https://web.archive.org/web/20240414151905/https:/www.artchive.com/artists/joseph-cornell/.

2 Doug Van Gundy, "Keeper," in *A Life Above Water: Poems* (Red Hen Press, 2007), 13.

I inverted my childhood fascination with fish and water; it was the trout who envied my life above water and not the other way around. "Keeper" also hints at the way a human fetus looks, in its early development, like an embryonic fish, and the way a fetus grows in a watery environment inside the womb. We are, through hundreds of millions of years of evolution, fish who have learned to live in the air.

The idea for the poem came to me in a flash, one day while fly-fishing the upper Williams River in West Virginia with my buddy Tim, a professional fly guide. I waded out of the water and laid my rod on the gravel bank to catch the poem in my notebook before it could wriggle away. I read my completed first draft to Tim, who had just released his fourth or fifth trout of the morning. When I finished, he asked me, "How do you think like that?" What I thought but didn't say was, *How do you not?* All of the elements of the poem lay at our feet all day—the limestone boulders, the brook trout and creek chubs, the caddis flies both real and fashioned from feathers and thread—why didn't he connect them into the lyric constellation I saw and heard?

Someone shared a brain teaser with me recently that is supposed to predict whether you are neurodivergent or neurotypical. She showed me a piece of cardstock with the characters "2" and "7" printed on it and asked me, "How are these alike?" Almost instantly, I answered: "They are both leaning to the right and both appear to be 'looking' to the left, they're similar in size and shape, and they are both black." She waited a beat before saying: "And they're both numbers."

The Scottish comedian Fern Brady, who is on the autism spectrum, describes neurotypical and neurodivergent brains as having two different operating systems, like Android phones and iPhones. The reason my buddy Tim didn't see a poem in gravel, dead sycamore leaves, and the play of sunlight through the water on the backs of the finning fish that day on the river is the same reason I've never been able to do the detailed work of fashioning an imitation insect from beads and bits of fur, the craft supplies that nearly come alive in Tim's hands. We have different operating systems.

*

I first encountered the concept of the *Wunderkammer* (literally "room of wonders") after I discovered Cornell. These "cabinets of curiosities," as they're called in English, were an inspiration to Cornell and are like his miniature constructions writ large: curated rooms of specimens, art, relics, and ephemera, gathered together without categorical distinction, simply because they are interesting. (Google "Joseph Cornell's basement studio," and you can find photographs of the collection of ephemera he drew from to create his remarkable constructions.)

Wunderkammern began appearing in the late sixteenth century in Europe as expressions of the Age of Discovery. As Europeans sailed to (and colonized) distant lands, they collected natural and ethnographic souvenirs: brilliantly colored butterflies, fish skeletons, African masks, pressed plants, Native American costumes and weapons, and much more. After returning home, they arranged and displayed their finds. In the late seventeenth and early eighteenth centuries, the discussion and study of such "oddities" was of both social and scientific importance. In such collections were the origins of some of the world's great natural history museums. In fact, the British Museum and the Natural History Museum in London both have their origins in the 1853 bequest of over 71,000 items from the personal collection of Sir Hans Sloane, an Anglo-Irish physician and naturalist who, among other things, is credited with the invention of chocolate milk.

(An aside: while fact-checking the spelling of *Wunderkammer* on Wikipedia—like YouTube, a cabinet of digital curiosities in its own right—I learned that the Ashmolean Museum at Oxford University was the first public museum in England, opening in 1683. The Ashmolean was built to house the collection of one Elias Ashmole, a wealthy collector of pretty much everything. In addition to its art, ethnography, and natural history collections, the Ashmolean houses the "Messiah" Stradivarius violin and the world's largest collection of astrolabes.)

Wunderkammern feel like a useful metaphor for the way my brain and memory work. It makes perfect sense to me that the raven's feather I found on a long-dead fiddler's grave in West Virginia and a stone I found by William Blake's tombstone would belong together, both in my mind and in the physical world. And why wouldn't the paper ticket from my first-ever ride on the Paris Métro and the stub from an R.E.M. show I saw in Salt Lake City in 1984 share drawer space with a palm-size photograph of a zeppelin floating above a farm field that I found at a flea market? Each is a memento of a significant first, a time when my mind was pried open just a little bit wider and the world was made just a little bit smaller.

The idea of the *Wunderkammer* helped me organize a collection of poems I had been working on. Over the course of a few years, I had written around a hundred poems that all seemed concerned with the importance of place and the influence of place on identity, and vice versa. I reread all these poems, then laid them neatly in rows on the living room floor. Once I had reconsidered each of the poems, I walked around the room in my stocking feet, trying to hear what they might be saying to one another. Several of the poems were saying nearly the same thing, so I placed those in a stack on the coffee table. Others didn't really seem to be talking to any of the other poems, or even to themselves. Those, too, joined the coffee-table reject pile. Eventually, I rejected over half of the poems, winnowing the number of candidate poems down to forty-nine. I rearranged the poems into groups I hoped might have that emergent property of meaning that Cornell's best pieces do. After some trial and error, I found there were three connected themes, and these became the three sections of the manuscript. The finished manuscript feels like a river to me, and the sections are different views of the river in different stages and moods, from different vantages. The individual poems feel like flat stones skipped across the surface of that river, never living completely in the water or the air.

In order for Cornell to make his singular art, it was important that he have much more ephemera and collectanea than he could ever possibly use. He also needed to be able to easily locate all that material. His basement studio was filled with repurposed cardboard cartons and folders labeled "Cordial Glasses," "Map Tacks," "Best White Boxes," "Stamps," et cetera. Like Cornell with his collections, I've had to develop organizational strategies, like keeping several journals at a time (one for writing, one for notes, a bullet journal, a reading journal) and maintaining an electronic calendar to send me reminders of events and deadlines. These practices have helped me make my collections less stressful and more useful. Medication has helped me put these strategies into practice.

But much of my collection lives inside my head as remembered facts and experiences, imagined lives, and parallel possible worlds where trout can talk. The more I'm able to think of my brain as a neurological *Wunderkammer*, the better I'm able to use it efficiently and the more joy I derive from its eclectic collections. The same qualities the Cornell shadow boxes helped me to embrace—impulsivity, shifting focus, a magpie-like tendency to collect objects and ideas—can be creative advantages.

I couldn't have written the aforementioned poem, "Keeper," which is scarcely a page in length, if I hadn't spent hundreds of hours on rivers and streams, alone and with my biologist father. I wouldn't have been able to visualize the development of the human fetus (and its more than passing resemblance to a fish embryo) if I hadn't spent hours poring over my mother's old nursing school anatomy books. And I wouldn't have been able to imagine the mind of a daydreaming trout if I hadn't devoted most of my life to being a daydreaming boy. The leaps and jumps I make in this poem and others begin in my mind, of course, but they are rarely unsupported. The breadth and depth of my interest in the world and the stickiness of my memory allow me to intuit where I'm going to land when I make that leap of language or imagery, even if it's the first time I've made the jump. My ricocheting ADHD brain and my ping-ponging poetry brain are one and the same.

*

In *Letters to a Young Poet*, Rainer Maria Rilke wrote: "And even if you were in some prison, the walls of which let none of the sounds of the world come to your senses—would you not then still have your childhood, that precious, kingly possession, that treasure-house of memories?"[3]

Now when I consider *my* treasure-house of childhood memories, I have nothing but tenderness for the weird boy who didn't quite fit in. I admire his boundless sense of wonder that was not dampened by (frankly impossible) expectations of conformity. That boy's delight lives inside me, along with every book I've ever read and every bleached bone I've ever found in the forest. My cluttered thoughts and leaps of imagination aren't distractions or obstacles. Like Cornell's boxes of cordial glasses and feathers, they are resources waiting to be used in my art.

3 Rainer Maria Rilke, *Letters to a Young Poet*, trans. Reginald Snell (Dover, 2002), 12.

PROMPT: Making Connections in the *Wunderkammer* of Your Mind

This prompt may not lead you to a finished draft, but it is an excellent prewriting exercise, especially for lyric essays and poems.

1. Fold a piece of paper in half lengthwise, then open it up again. On the left side of the paper, list ten of your interests or obsessions. On the right side, list ten specific objects you own or have collected that are fascinating or important to you.
2. Divide another sheet of paper into a 4 × 5 grid (20 boxes). Distribute the words from the two lists you just made among the boxes at random, one word per box.
3. This step is very important! Put the grid away for *at least two hours*—or better yet, a day or three.
4. When you can't stand to wait any longer, return to your grid. Read each word aloud. How are the words in dialogue with each other? How do they connect narratively? Emotionally? Thematically? Chronologically? Do they speak to each other in more ways than one?
5. Start exploring the connections among these juxtaposed interests and objects in your writing.

DOUGLAS KEARNEY

4

I began doing type experiments because I was interested in simultaneity and I have said this before and am always saying it even when I am not doing type experiments then the type is the performed absence of simultaneity I mean to mean a discipline of singularity I've discussed discipline before and here's what I said

discipline (as in métier) (as in correction)

so I am thinking graphically enacting simultaneity there is no text behind the box because I mean to be legible right now no I mean to signal *signal* optically even as syntactically I am threatening noise when I realized my legibility as such which is to say to those who wish to noise my signal can say I signal noise which isn't a contradiction though contradiction is fine because *contradiction* as not allowed is dribbling a basketball with two hands as in against the rules but in a game in which you can dribble with either hand I began playing basketball when I was but I don't mean to mean that I been playing basketball for a long time even as I mean to mean on some *who sees me as signal of noise which is to noise my signal* though I suppose recipients been making signal noise or signal and noise signal or noise but I also mean to mean I could also mean to mean that those who noise me aren't intended recipients of my signal or my noise a basketball intercepted when passed at which point the ball hyper-legible to the recipients who weren't recipients a signal hypo-legibile so much is happening simultaneously and simultaneously how I mean to read this aloud and not the armor poems trying to be multiple signals simultaneously noises my body a noise that noises the poem as visual signals into noise by way of translation and translation simultaneous signal and noise and I don't mean to mean to noise my body either because it cannot hold the multiplicitous signals simultaneously or because I don't mean to mean to signal my body noise what renders its signal noise and I only know how to do that by not staying doing what I been stayed doing by way of turning an idea into type a visual signal of sound here the sound stay doing somewhere not me but signaled as me simultaneously as opposed to here where we are now where simultaneity stay hypo-legible even as all this type here is here but by way of multiplicity you probably making signal dear recipient taking signal dear recipient one word at a time because you disciplined ain't you dear recipient disciplined dear recipient ain't you (as in métier) (as in correction)

???

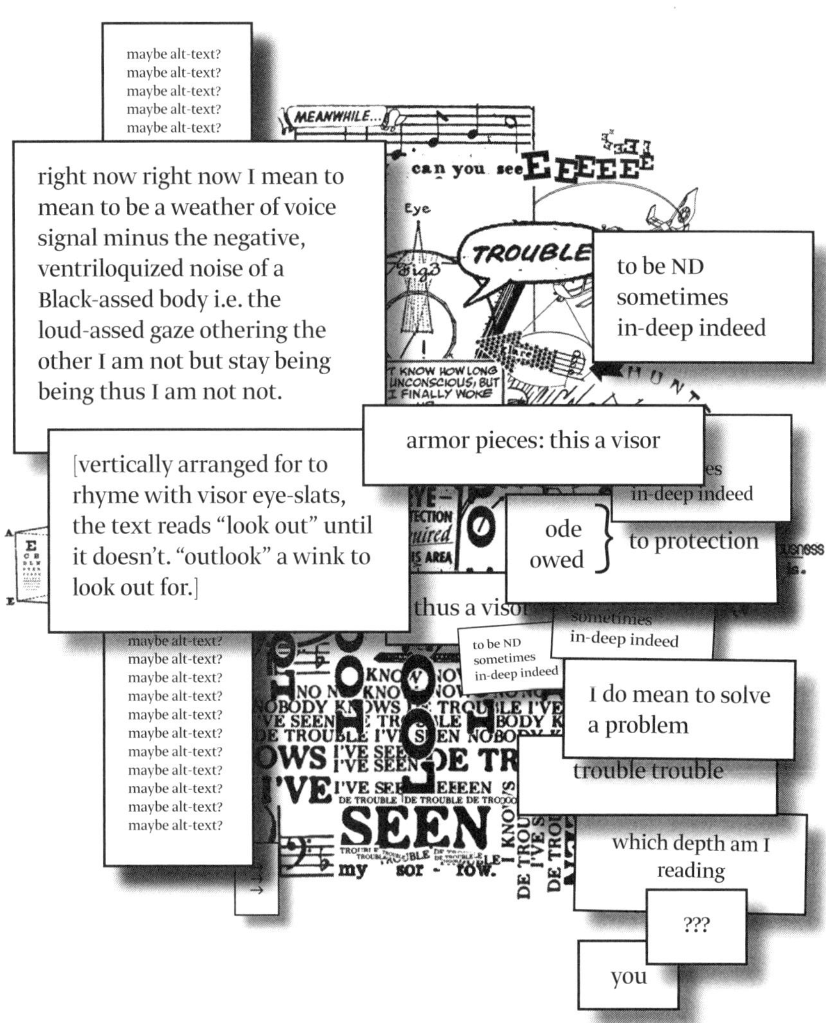
maybe alt-text?
maybe alt-text?
maybe alt-text?
maybe alt-text?
maybe alt-text?
MEANWHILE...
can you seeEEEEE
right now right now I mean to mean to be a weather of voice signal minus the negative, ventriloquized noise of a Black-assed body i.e. the loud-assed gaze othering the other I am not but stay being being thus I am not not.
Eye
TROUBLE
to be ND
sometimes
in-deep indeed
I KNOW HOW LONG UNCONSCIOUS, BUT I FINALLY WOKE
armor pieces: this a visor
[vertically arranged for to rhyme with visor eye-slats, the text reads "look out" until it doesn't. "outlook" a wink to look out for.]
in-deep indeed
ode
owed
to protection
thus a visor
sometimes
in-deep indeed
to be ND
sometimes
in-deep indeed
maybe alt-text?
maybe alt-text?
maybe alt-text?
maybe alt-text?
maybe alt-text?
maybe alt-text?
maybe alt-text?
maybe alt-text?
maybe alt-text?
maybe alt-text?
maybe alt-text?
I do mean to solve
a problem
trouble trouble
NOBODY KNOWS DE TROUBLE I'VE SEEN
SEEN
my sor - row.
which depth am I
reading
???
you

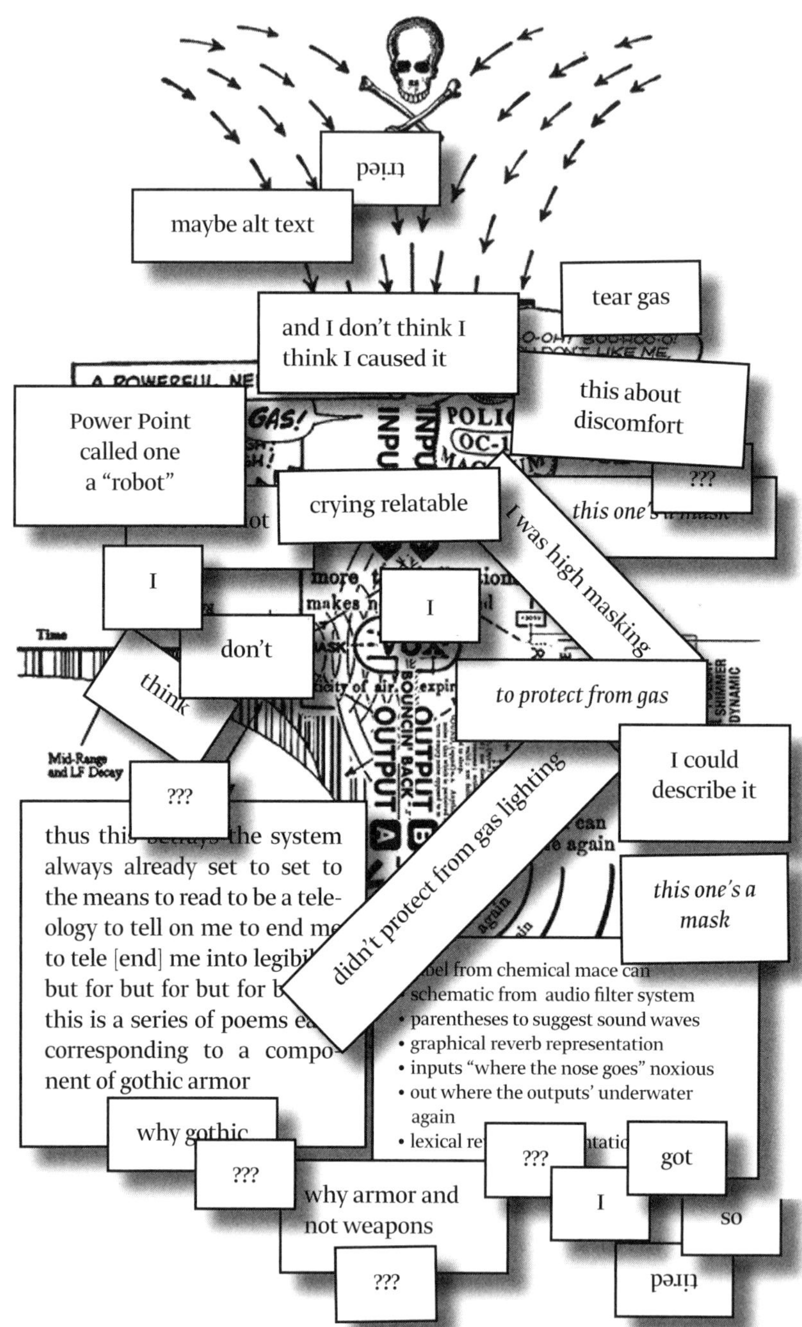
tried
maybe alt text
tear gas
and I don't think I think I caused it
this about discomfort
Power Point called one a "robot"
crying relatable
???
this one's a mask
I was high masking
I
I
don't
think
to protect from gas
Time
Mid-Range and LF Decay
???
I could describe it
didn't protect from gas lighting
thus this betrays the system always already set to set to the means to read to be a teleology to tell on me to end me to tele [end] me into legibility but for but for but for b
this is a series of poems each corresponding to a component of gothic armor
this one's a mask
• label from chemical mace can
• schematic from audio filter system
• parentheses to suggest sound waves
• graphical reverb representation
• inputs "where the nose goes" noxious
• out where the outputs' underwater again
• lexical representation
why gothic
???
why armor and not weapons
???
???
I
got
so
tried

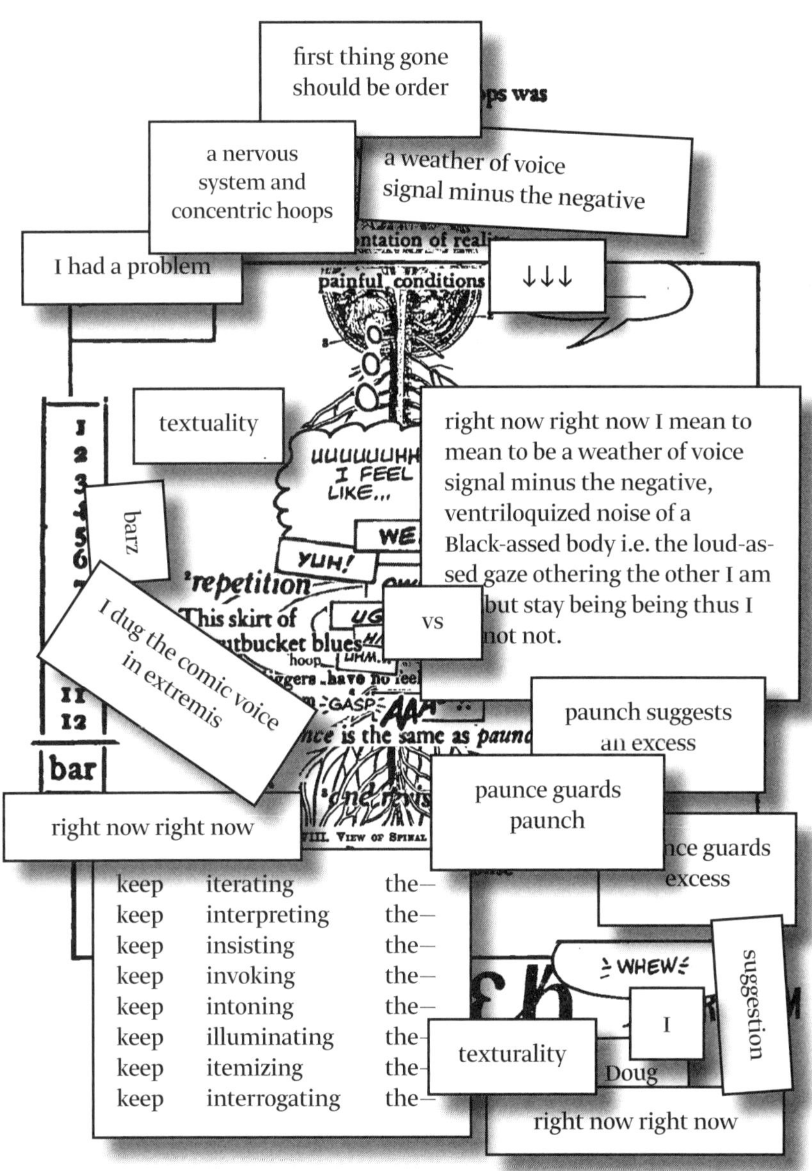
first thing gone
should be order
ps was
a nervous
system and
concentric hoops
a weather of voice
signal minus the negative
I had a problem
painful conditions
↓↓↓
textuality
UUUUUUHH
I FEEL
LIKE...
barz
WE
YUH!
right now right now I mean to
mean to be a weather of voice
signal minus the negative,
ventriloquized noise of a
Black-assed body i.e. the loud-assed gaze othering the other I am
but stay being being thus I
not not.
repetition
This skirt of
utbucket blues
vs
I dug the comic voice
in extremis
GASP
nce is the same as paun
11
12
bar
paunch suggests
an excess
paunce guards
paunch
right now right now
nce guards
excess
keep iterating the—
keep interpreting the—
keep insisting the—
keep invoking the—
keep intoning the—
keep illuminating the—
keep itemizing the—
keep interrogating the—
WHEW
I
suggestion
texturality
Doug
right now right now

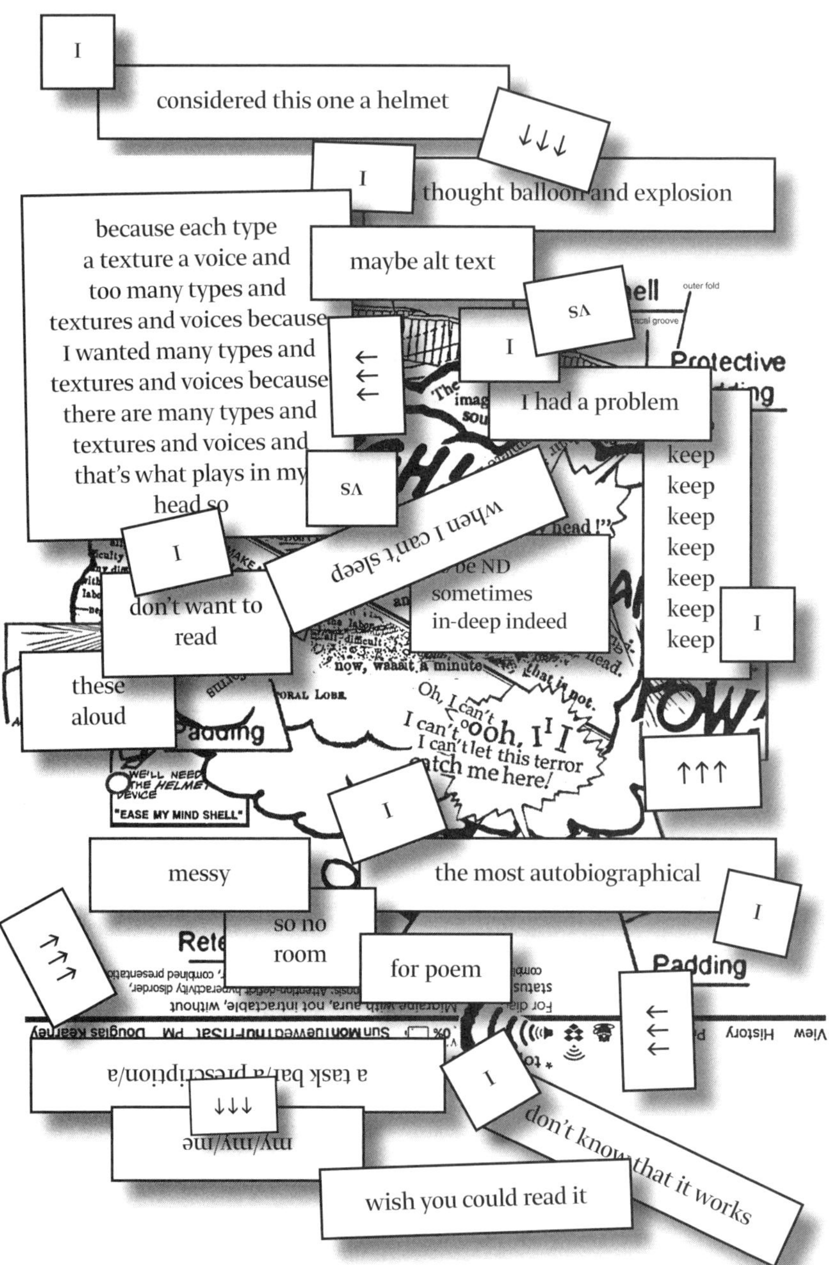
I
considered this one a helmet
↓↓↓
I
thought balloon and explosion
because each type
a texture a voice and
too many types and
textures and voices because
I wanted many types and
textures and voices because
there are many types and
textures and voices and
that's what plays in my
head so
maybe alt text
vs
←←←
I
I had a problem
Protective
outer fold
keep
keep
keep
keep
keep
keep
keep
I
vs
when I can't sleep
I
don't want to
read
be ND
sometimes
in-deep indeed
these
aloud
Oh, I can't
I can't ooh, I I I
I can't let this terror
catch me here!
now, waaait, a minute
"EASE MY MIND SHELL"
↑↑↑
I
messy
the most autobiographical
I
↑↑↑
so no
room
for poem
Padding
←←←
a task bar/a prescription/a
↓↓↓
my/my/me
I
don't know that it works
wish you could read it

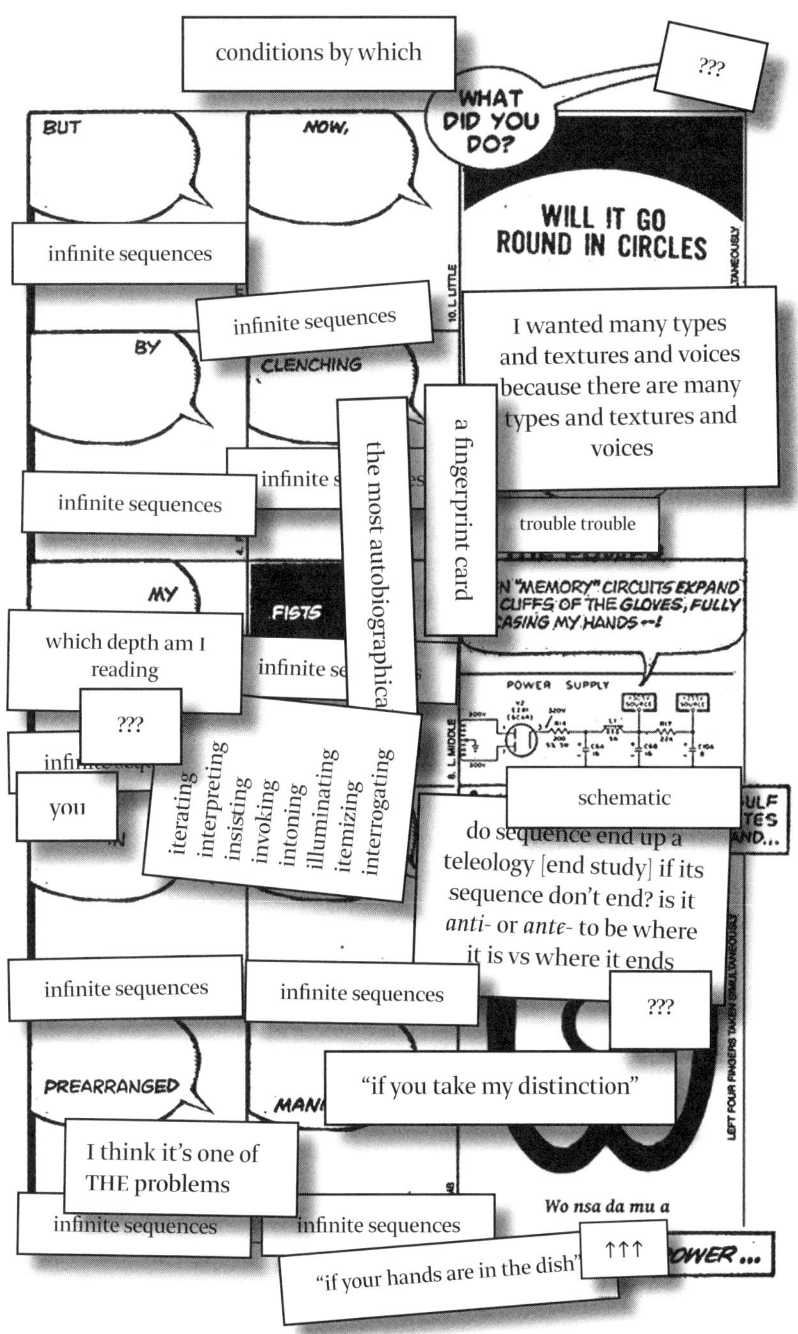
conditions by which
???
WHAT DID YOU DO?
BUT
NOW,
WILL IT GO ROUND IN CIRCLES
infinite sequences
infinite sequences
I wanted many types and textures and voices because there are many types and textures and voices
BY
CLENCHING
the most autobiographical
a fingerprint card
infinite sequences
trouble trouble
MY
FISTS
"MEMORY" CIRCUITS EXPAND CUFFS OF THE GLOVES, FULLY CASING MY HANDS--!
which depth am I reading
???
POWER SUPPLY
iterating
interpreting
insisting
invoking
intoning
illuminating
itemizing
interrogating
you
schematic
do sequence end up a teleology [end study] if its sequence don't end? is it *anti-* or *ante-* to be where it is vs where it ends
infinite sequences
infinite sequences
???
PREARRANGED
"if you take my distinction"
I think it's one of THE problems
infinite sequences
infinite sequences
Wo nsa da mu a
"if your hands are in the dish"
↑↑↑
LEFT FOUR FINGERS TAKEN SIMULTANEOUSLY

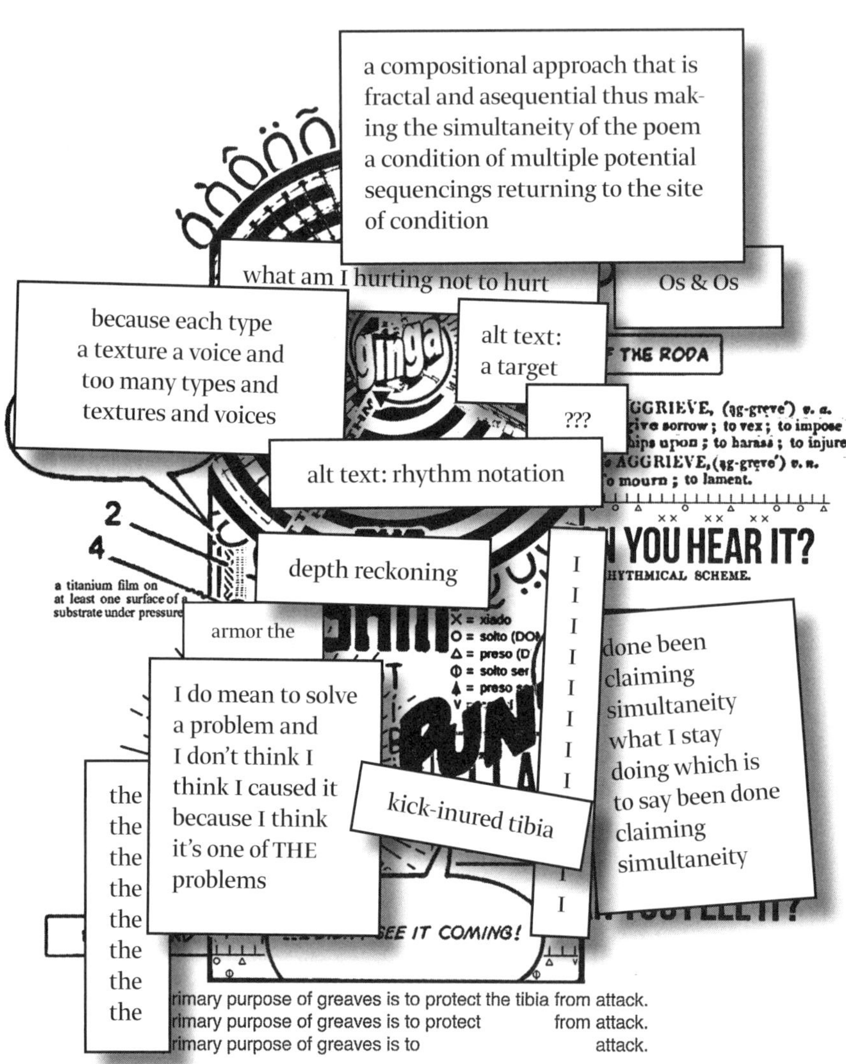
a compositional approach that is fractal and asequential thus making the simultaneity of the poem a condition of multiple potential sequencings returning to the site of condition
what am I hurting not to hurt
Os & Os
because each type a texture a voice and too many types and textures and voices
ginga
alt text: a target
THE RODA
???
AGGRIEVE, (ag-greve') v. a. give sorrow; to vex; to impose hips upon; to harass; to injure.
AGGRIEVE, (ag-greve') v. n. to mourn; to lament.
alt text: rhythm notation
2
4
YOU HEAR IT?
RHYTHMICAL SCHEME.
depth reckoning
a titanium film on at least one surface of a substrate under pressure
armor the
X = xiado
O = solto (DO
Δ = preso (D
Φ = solto se
= preso
I
I
I
I
I
I
I
I
I
I
done been claiming simultaneity what I stay doing which is to say been done claiming simultaneity
I do mean to solve a problem and I don't think I think I caused it because I think it's one of THE problems
kick-inured tibia
the
the
the
the
the
the
the
the
SEE IT COMING!
rimary purpose of greaves is to protect the tibia from attack.
rimary purpose of greaves is to protect from attack.
rimary purpose of greaves is to attack.

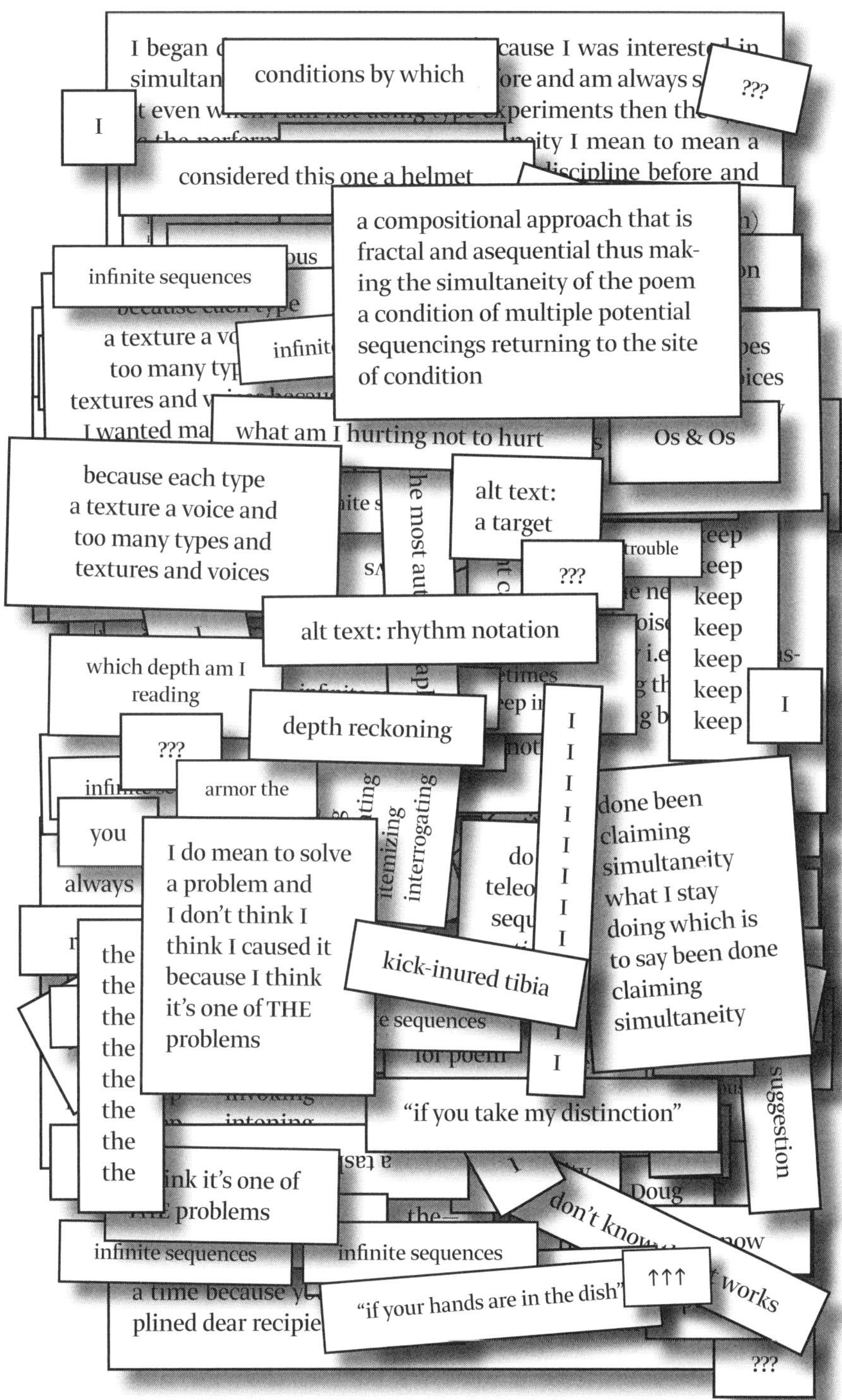
conditions by which
???
I
considered this one a helmet
a compositional approach that is fractal and asequential thus making the simultaneity of the poem a condition of multiple potential sequencings returning to the site of condition
infinite sequences
what am I hurting not to hurt
Os & Os
because each type a texture a voice and too many types and textures and voices
alt text: a target
trouble
???
keep keep keep keep keep keep keep
alt text: rhythm notation
which depth am I reading
depth reckoning
I
???
armor the
itemizing
interrogating
I I I I I I I I I I I
done been claiming simultaneity what I stay doing which is to say been done claiming simultaneity
you
always
I do mean to solve a problem and I don't think I think I caused it because I think it's one of THE problems
kick-inured tibia
the the the the the the the the
"if you take my distinction"
suggestion
Doug
infinite sequences
infinite sequences
"if your hands are in the dish"
↑↑↑
???

5

Anything I Fix My Mind To

On Process and Embracing Change

KWOYA FAGIN MAPLES

First, y'all, a poem:

Attention Deficit Pastoral

Or how, if there is field before me—broad sky,
and too much green—I lose my breath,
forgetting.
Unable to keep up with my body,
now lifted off to wonder.
My children knock
around my knees, yet I can't hear their pulling.
So much is stunning me at once, the sun
on me at once. Why this?
I go in blind direction
smelling woods or earth or air,
so many roads of grass
under my shoes.[1]

Space-Cadet. Careless. Daydreamer. And the one that gets under my skin the most: *Weird*. Even with my best attempts at masking, there are slips of my offbeat, just off-step-ness, that are impossible to miss.

1 Kwoya Fagin Maples, "Attention Deficit Pastoral" © 2019 by Kwoya Fagin Maples. First appeared on *Tin House Online*, November 20, 2019.

For example: while highly sensitive to the faintest repetitive sound, I am rarely startled by loud or unexpected noises. My mind, full and distracting, turns down the volume of those around me with and without my consent.

Another example: my inner monologue is persistent, always rewording and shifting language—even during conversations that are rather important. This isn't selective listening; that creative voice is often louder and I've practiced listening to it more than others. I'm afraid I'll miss something, especially in the process of writing a book. Like most writers, I exist between creativity and daily experiences (and I live *for* heightened experiences). For my brain, this can be (pleasurably) overwhelming. Sometimes my cognitive experience is like a swinging door between the outside world and disassociation, like the moment of being "lifted off to wonder" I describe in the poem. The swinging door refers to the ease with which my mind shifts focus from the external (family, friends, conversation) to the internal (writing, wordplay, emotion). It's difficult to pull myself out of wonder when I'm stuck in it because my brain has been seeking something stimulating to fall into.

This can be good for my writing, but it can pose challenges. When drafting a poem, my thoughts may arrive unordered, in more of an "and this, and this, + that" association, until my internal critic interrupts with cries of *Order!* But what is the "right order" for these lines, anyway? Sometimes when I don't understand my own transitions, I *over*-overcorrect by googling "poetic structure," and before I know it I'm looking at forest-green braiding hair on Amazon for my next hair appointment. When I pick up the poem's threads again, I experience a moment of panic because I am afraid I won't be able to remember the subtleties of the poem. The logic is often reflective of the moment I was writing it. With my reliance on artistic/external influences of the moment, the connections may seem weak, the references obscure.

When I am at my best as a writer, I draft the language in the poem based on external observation. I commit to the words and moves as they come. I enjoy witnessing how my brain moves with imagination that is uninhibited. One of my consistently successful techniques for writing poems is to sit in a public place and write as ideas occur based on my location. I may start with an idea related to personal experience, but I am ultra-friendly with the swinging door, allowing off-subject associative ideas and images from the environment into the poem as they arise: pieces of conversation, people, and animals. I consider this a *mode* of writing. For me, this is the way that writing feels most reflexive. In revision, my task then becomes resisting over-editing, explanation, and the internal "ordering police." *I must protect the imagination of the work*. With these poems, I make a decision to not allow myself to fundamentally change the work. It's a practice of being faithful: to myself, to the moment, to the way my mind moves. When I protect the imagination of my work, I get the most pleasure out of reading it later, to myself or to an audience. The poems I've written this way seem to connect the most with other people, and they are the writing I am most proud of.

What I love most about the way my brain works is that it allows me to hyperfocus through immersion. Immersive topics—I call them "wells"—allow me to engage intellectually, somatically, and sensorily with the material. Not only is this pleasurable for me as an artist, but it is my strategy for remaining engaged, whether completing writing projects or designing a class. Often, my motivation is directly connected to what is most exciting and stimulating to me. My experience of every art form feeds that need for consumption. My brain has a sweet tooth and I overindulge. I resent boredom, so I try to add a treat whenever I have to complete a dull task: time at a café, "body doubling" by working alongside a friend, or allowing myself to indulge in procrastination. Sometimes a combination of all of these.

For writing, I often seek those "wells" by choosing projects with depth—endless research paths through history, visual art, and musical forms. Choosing these kinds of projects allows me to engage deeply with my work once I find a *purpose*—usually by connecting the project to those who came before me, my ancestors. On my mom's side, I was a second-generation college student. On my dad's, I was first generation. I came from a family with several military members and blue-collar workers. I still struggle with poetry's place in my life. Having a larger purpose satisfies that hardworking/grit mentality I was socialized with. Like it or lump it, purpose becomes the voice that pushes me throughout the process of writing a book. Immersive, wondrous experiences become the fodder, the sweet spots that foster creativity and make writing pleasurable. Finding purpose encourages my motivation to continue (and fully complete) the project.

My first book-length collection, *Mend* (University Press of Kentucky, 2018), tells the story of the birth of gynecology and the role that Black enslaved women played in that process. Dr. James Marion Sims began a series of experiments on these women between 1845 and 1849. My book tells the story from the women's points of view. It is written in historical persona, in the voices of the women.

In 2018, I began my third book-length project, *Long Eye* (Hub City Press, 2026). Primarily, the work is oceanic and autobiographical. I am from Charleston, South Carolina, and the Atlantic Ocean serves as a touchstone, the link between my childhood and adulthood. Because I consider purpose, I thought of my ancestors and their connection to the Atlantic, which would become the heart of the project. As I set out to write this book, I didn't have a fixed process or plan, but I knew that (1) I would have to find ways to engage the reader outside of my own personal experience; (2) I would need a plan for producing new poems when I didn't feel like writing; (3) I would utilize immersive practices.

The process that emerged was uniquely suited to my brain and my way of working. I want to lay out that process and the book's chronological development here:

1. *Setting a practice intention*: When I set my writing goals for 2018, I decided that I wanted to write two new poems per week. It didn't matter whether the writing was strong or not. It was more about keeping the practice. I shared this goal with my husband so he'd be on board with covering more of our household needs, and so he'd hold me accountable (even if I procrastinated until Sunday night). To feed my creative brain, I decided to read at least one poetry collection a week and respond to it. The result was that I drafted two poems per week. At least one poem was a response, especially during weeks I didn't *feel* like writing. Since this plan was my own (and not copied from a Pinterest board), I was actually able to follow it. I practiced this approach for eight months.
2. *Atmospheric intentionality/choosing a space to write into*: I'm often intentional about *where* I write to optimize my attention and enhance my creative work—not just geographically, but atmospherically. For an immersive and sensory experience during this project, I began the practice of writing on shorelines of the Atlantic over a period of four years. I wrote from chairs I'd set near the surf, the water flooding my feet. Or I picked up my pen right after a swim, droplets wetting my notebook. Since my subject was as old as writing itself, I was highly concerned with accuracy and originality. The sensory experience of being on the beach allowed me both. I thought of fresh ideas for word choices, for ways of describing my own experiences with the ocean. Since I began to notice more, I also considered my social interactions on the beach as a person of color, and these experiences made it into the poems.
3. *Embracing a soundscape*: In addition to reading companion books, I passively listened to books about tidal patterns. I listened while I braided my daughters' hair or as I commuted, or even as I fell asleep. This is because (like Mrs. Jewls and Sharie in *Sideways Stories from Wayside School*) I believe in learning by osmosis. It is okay for my mind to wander or sleep. What I want is to experience language. The auditory experience produces images and fills your word bank. Listening without pressure to understand is

a relief, a mental break from more arduous forms of research. It gives my brain a sense of accomplishment, and I believe that all those words are now up there in the cloud (as it were), waiting to be downloaded when needed.

4. *Finding a physical practice connected to the project*: I took my first set of lessons and finally learned how to swim. I swam across a pool for the first time while writing this book, then I swam in the ocean. I wanted to learn how to give my body to water and know I wouldn't sink. I wanted to be able to describe the feel and pull of water more accurately. I took lessons with a kind instructor who also became my daughters' instructor. I swam at least twice a week for months, either with my instructor or alone at the Y. My body felt strong. It built my faith in my body's capacity and reaffirmed my resolve to remain a lifelong learner, to stay open to learning new things. Looking back, it was one of the highlights of this project.
5. *Doing historical research*: After I finished the personal poems, I wanted to add what I call "the third thing" to the manuscript. The third thing, for me, is often a poetic series, which can become the spine of the collection and is perhaps what ultimately attracts the reader to the book. For my third thing, I decided to situate the personal within the historical. I began to look at history related to Black Americans and the ocean. While researching, I came across an 1803 mass suicide that took place at Igbo Landing, near St. Simons Island, Georgia. It was at this site that at least thirteen enslaved people attempted to drown themselves rather than face life with their traffickers. This story is what led me to learn about the water spirit/mermaid who some of these people believed would take them home. In West African religion, Mami Wata lives in every body of water. Her role is to care for the needy who approach the water and to lead lost souls to the afterlife. This mermaid would ultimately appear in a series of poems that became a central part of the manuscript.
6. *Creating a writing retreat*: By October 2022, I'd decided to draft a long poem in the voice of a mermaid. After much contemplating

and research, the poem was arriving. It had taken months to get to this point. I cleared my schedule and used research funds to travel to Igbo Landing at St. Simons Island. I felt I needed the sensory experience of immersion, so I followed my instincts. I went there to physically stand near the site and speculate, to write at the water's edge in the mornings, and to work late into the night at my hotel until my thinking dulled, my eyes blurred, and I was terribly hungry. Waking up to deer standing in front of the ocean is an image I won't forget. This immersive isolation was what allowed me to focus and write in the final stages of the manuscript—it was also a way for me to wield my ability to hyperfocus as a useful tool in the journey to completion. While writing *Mend* I made a similar trip, traveling to Mount Meigs, Alabama, to the land where the doctor's house was. I was unable to find the exact location of his house; the directions I was given by a local historian led me to an abandoned cotton field. The book ended up including poems about the process of trying to find the doctor's house, as well as poems about the historian, who I renamed Mary Catherine. I know that I will continue to rely on these kinds of immersive processes in the future. It's my favorite thing about being a writer.

7. *Putting it together, sending it out*: I picked a poetry manuscript submission deadline that would generate a sense of urgency: *Now I have 31 days*. I worked with a writing coach to help me develop a final revision plan and checked in with her regularly for accountability. In the final month before the deadline, I worked for several hours most days. I organized the poems and completed final edits to produce a completed manuscript and sent it off. When I accomplished my goal, I went on Instagram and posted photos of my messy office and a video my daughter captured of my victory dance.

None of the steps of this process were clear to me at the outset. I see it all now, in retrospect.

*

I have never been a writer who writes every day. I've been writing (professionally) for at least twenty years. Early on, I didn't accept this about myself. I have learned, however, that writing in intensive shorter bursts is best for me. In times of overwhelm, I get work done and preserve space for writing by keeping a loose form of "priority/block scheduling" (*loose*, because anything more structured induces guilt, stress, and won't become a habit). Right now, Wednesdays are for teaching and conferencing with students, and Mondays are heavy "admin" days for me. On Fridays, I get caught up on things around the house. Thursdays are supposed to be the days I read and grade. Despite medication, vitamins, exercise, positivity, spiritual connectedness, and prayer, there is a day each week when my brain needs rest from executive tasks. More often than not, I give my brain that rest on Thursday and catch up on that grading later, somehow.

Since I am often routine resistant, all of this is subject to change. I have decided, however, that *writing and creativity are my important things*. Writing and creativity are what feed and motivate me, what give me the energy and focus to do the other stuff. Some semesters I have a scheduled writing day. As in, I schedule nothing else on that day and preserve it for writing. Often, it's Tuesday. My brain likes the letters in the word Tuesday; it reminds me of the number two, its perfection, and makes me think of art. If I want to get writing done, a coffee shop is best, others working beside me holding me accountable (and as I write this essay I'm at a café, though now my fingers have become cold and I'll need to leave soon to begin my hour-long commute to teach a course I've titled "From Stars to Constellation: Structures of the Poetry Collection"). Once I actually *feel* like writing and am able to start, I'm afraid to stop. A lot of us have to take advantage of bursts of energy to accomplish tasks because we don't know how long the bursts will last. (When I say *us*, I mean other ADHDers, instead of my usual use of *Us* for other Black people.)

I love organizational systems. I research planners (obsessively), find the best one in the world, purchase it, and then barely use it. Or I use it for a while before moving on to something else. Same goes for various apps, lists, whiteboards, and family calendars. This switching between systems is particularly hard on my neurotypical, Type-A husband. I wasn't diagnosed until we'd lived together for seven years. I blamed my inattentiveness, anxiety, and forgetfulness on *being an artist*. After fourteen years, now we understand that in order for me to stay organized, I actually need to regularly change how I stay organized and productive. My writing practices don't change much. However, the practice of intentionally reading and writing in response, which I began while writing my current collection, has stuck around. It helped me read more new books and generate more new work than I typically would have. It also produced accountability for me as a mother and professor, reminding me to prioritize writing.

*

> I go in blind direction
> smelling woods or earth or air,
> so many roads of grass
> under my shoes.

My mind sends me down such cool pathways—I'm theorizing, writing award-winning books, woodworking, painting, making shopping lists for my family. And sometimes I'm just daydreaming. And no, that doesn't mean I'm not working: I have a job that pays me to be a daydreamer, teaching creative writing at the University of Alabama.

Many times, I have been annoyed, dismayed, and angry with myself. But I have to accept my brain—love it, even—and the people closest to me are allowed to be irritated or frustrated, but they, too, have to accept my brain. They have to be willing to tell me, like my husband, Marcus, that "ADHD is a superpower." Since he's a huge Marvel fan, it made me tear up the first time he said it. I was diagnosed as an adult at thirty-four. In terms of severity/impact, I've scored at least a nine on a ten-point scale. Like a lot of folks, it was a struggle for me to accept the diagnosis—still is, and it's been seven years since then.

I couldn't write this essay without acknowledging the difficult and frustrating effects of ADHD. They exist. But when I talk with newly diagnosed folks who are discouraged and feel that they aren't "true" writers because of their symptoms, I share my own experiences. I am a mother of three elementary-aged children. I am a writer, professor, and woodworker (I build bookshelves). Managing all of this "adulting," as Gen Z says, is not easy.

If true writers have an Excel spreadsheet of submissions and write every day, what am I? I am *this kind* of order: I write slowly, but I savor the process. I linger. I commit and fall deeply into my work. What if the way we do things is already enough? Through a neurotypical lens, the one we all hold up, it's disordered, but, reader, however you write, it's *your way*. And it works. What finally changed for me was prioritizing acceptance and validating *how I already choose* to go about things. This is order. I am order. Maybe we don't need to finally incorporate that TikTok-worthy "morning, afternoon, and nighttime routine." Maybe we begin to *notice* what circumstances most encourage us to pursue art.

A Few Tips for Immersive Writing

- When possible, travel to the location you will be writing about. This provides fresh and unique sensory details beyond your imagination and memory. Visual artists are told to "draw what they see and not what they know." A writer immersed in the environment of their subject has access to additional opportunities for accuracy, influence, and surprise.
- A lack of information doesn't mean a stopping point for the work. It means you have to approach research more creatively. For *Mend*, I read slave narratives collected by the WPA in the 1930s. I printed out photographs and pinned them up around the space

I wrote in, and I wrote while listening to music from that time period. In particular, music helped me develop a voice for the collection and consider the women's outlook and motivations. I also incorporated some of the lyrics into my poems as found text.

- For longer projects, consider separating research time from writing time. This leaves room for imagination and creativity and gives the work some space from the research. I researched my first book for a year before I began writing.
- Try out ekphrasis (writing about visual art) and respond to the visual in your creative work. Using photos of the setting/people/objects you're writing about can be another way to access them if you can't interact with them in person.
- Incorporate found text from documents. Use direct quotes. Be willing to play with the language found as part of your process of investigation. What lines from a book on Floridian trees might be useful in your story set in Orlando? What suppositions might arise from a single sentence? Use language as a starting point, for example, by writing stream of consciousness or in the Zuihitsu form.

PROMPT: A Memory, a Story, a Song

1. Think of one of the most memorable stories from your childhood.
2. Reach out to a family member who tells that story best. After asking for their consent to record your conversation and use the material in a creative piece, have them recount the story. Ask follow-up questions to encourage them to expound on the story.
3. Search online for a song that reminds you of this story and listen to it.
4. Write a poem or short story that draws on both the interview and the song. Consider directly incorporating words, phrases, and images from the interview and/or the song into your creative piece. How has this story, or the telling of it, impacted who you've become?

6

The Third Word Is Shame

ROBIN BLACK

What I think of first when asked what ADHD has meant to me:
My childhood.

What I see first when I think of my childhood:
The floor of my bedroom, covered in dirty clothes, scraps of paper, random toy parts, food wrappers, stuffed animals, books, Magic Markers without their caps . . .

What I remember of my mother teasing the enormous snarls out of my hair:
Physical pain
    (Shame)

How my hair got like that:
It literally never occurred to me to brush it. It never occurred to me to do anything with any regularity.

What memory I associate with the word "shower":
Being in the girls' locker room in fifth grade and being certain that Ellie F. saying that *anyone who doesn't shower every day is just gross* was directed at me.

How often I showered in fifth grade:
Every few days. I guess. I have no idea. A far cry from every day. Maybe once a week. I don't know. There was no pattern to it, no consistency.

I don't really do consistency. I never have.

How many meanings the word "teasing" has:
At least two. Though as I sat there on the floor, my mother in the chair behind me with a comb, and I thought about kids making fun of my tangled hair, those meanings seemed to merge into one.

The first three words I associate with my childhood:
Hopeless. Weepy.

That's only two words . . .
The thing about shame is, it never goes away. When I was in graduate school, forty-one years old, I wrote a story that included a description of "bottles of beer in the refrigerator, tipped in among the lettuce and a packet of chicken breasts."

My advisor's margin comment: "But you don't keep lettuce and chicken in the same part of the fridge."

This took me aback. I had no idea. Don't you just shove things in where they fit? Or if they don't fit, turn them over in some way so they do fit—more or less? And if turning them over makes for spills, well, isn't that just how refrigerators work? You clean the spills after a few weeks, or months, often when you need to make room for some occasion, like maybe Thanksgiving.

Isn't that the quintessential householder/refrigerator relationship?

Apparently not.

How much of this I find amusing:
So close to none that I might as well say none.

None.

Really, none?
Well, there's this one story about an ancient roast beef sandwich tumbling out of my handbag onto the counter of a store so elegant it was pretty much a holy shrine to high fashion. Even I can laugh at that one.

My Life Story:
Once upon a time, there was a little girl named Robin. She was terrible at everything except reading. The End.

The long version:
Once upon a time, there was a little girl named Robin. She was terrible at everything, except reading. Reading was different because when she read, when she immersed herself in a story, she wasn't only escaping a world that felt overwhelming and poorly suited to her—a world of lost mittens, unbrushed teeth, late homework, and social awkwardness—she was also *entering* a world in which she felt capable, and interested, and in which she felt insightful.

And insight, it turned out, was the one thing she could do better than pretty much anyone she knew. (Perhaps they were all too busy *achieving* to really think through the more elusive points of human nature.) It might have felt like bragging for her to think that, even quietly to herself, but having spent her whole life aware only of how much she did poorly, this felt more like a consolation prize—or possibly more like a glimmer of hope.

Maybe, just maybe, the fact of understanding why people do the things they do, and seeing unusual connectors between their interior lives and their actions, finding those insights more interesting than anything else, could be something on which a person who had failed at pretty much everything involving the physical world might build a life . . .

How My Life Story ends:
And so with this new understanding of her own strengths, she pulled

herself together, began writing novels, and found peace and self-confidence at a very young age. The End.

Just kidding!

Why it wasn't close to that simple:

We associate so much of what is difficult for people with ADHD with character—in the most oppressive meaning of that word. Messy people are *slovenly*. Kids who never turn in their homework are *lazy*. Youngsters whose hair is an impenetrable tangle are just plain *disgusting*. Children whose rooms are filthy are *disobedient*. And—because I never outgrew much of it—mothers whose homes are filthy are suspect in any number of ways. People who don't pay their bills on time, people who don't get thank-you notes out, people who forget to return phone calls. And then there are the missed social cues, the not quite getting it, the saying the wrong thing . . .

In the absence of anything else to call it, a child naturally becomes convinced that they are definingly *wrong*. So, even though I began to realize that I was decent at piecing together clues about human nature, and recognized that I could sometimes have perceptive, clear thoughts, I still knew in my heart that I was a shameful person.

When I wrote my college application essays:

The night before they were due. I wrote them out longhand, off the top of my head, kind of crunching the words in at the bottom. God help me, I think they were in pencil.

I didn't know any better. I'm not sure it would have mattered if I had.

Why I am dwelling on the bad:

If I am to write about having ADHD, I need to be honest about the painful parts. I need to shine a light on the shame it caused me. Because fighting that shame is an enormous part of why I write.

The paradox of people with ADHD writing fiction:

Arguably, the last career for someone with this reflexive level of shame is writing. Never mind all the adjacent, organizational tasks for which ADHD leaves you profoundly unqualified—I am picturing those half-written submission letters on my bedroom floor, back in the day—writing requires that you be willing to endure endless, uncontrollable self-exposure. And this is truer of fiction than of memoir, counterintuitive though that may be. When I write an essay about myself, I choose what to tell and what to hold back. Having read this essay to this point, you know about the rat's nest hair and the unclean clothes, but who knows what shame-producing events occurred in my youth, or in my middle age, that are still too embarrassing for me to share? (I *may* know; you definitely *don't* know.)

Memoir, which is, by definition, an act of self-revelation, is equally an exercise in self-invention.

While fiction is something altogether else. Writing fiction, sharing it, is akin to showing your sleeping dreams to strangers. Embedded in all of our fictional works are our unexamined obsessions, our understanding of human behavior, our values, our oddities of perception and personality. Our strengths and our failings.

It's said that all authors write the same story again and again and again. As I understand that phenomenon, as I live it, it doesn't refer to anything like plot or characters, but rather to the fact that the preoccupations of the author remain the same from piece to piece, and can be unearthed by a canny reader.

There is little one can legally do in public that is as exposing as sharing one's own fictional visions.

A note about exposure:
I cook all the family holiday meals. I'm a really, really good cook. In fact, cooking was probably the second thing that I knew I could do well—after reading.

But I have come of age as a cook in the era of open kitchens, open-concept living. For decades, I have lived in homes with kitchens that double as the room where everyone gathers before the meal. And I hate it. Not when it's my immediate family—they are well-versed in all my most trying aspects. But when there are cousins, and in-laws, and whatever strays we may have welcomed in, I hate it. I do not want these people to see the chaos in which I operate. (I hate it.) The unwashed pots, about to fall from their stacks. The unwiped spills. (I *hate* it.) The lost pot holders I am cursing about.

I dread both the critical thoughts my guests are surely having, and the jokes they occasionally make. I want to be invisible while I cook. I want them all to go away. My mess is private. My failings are private. My shame is my business.

I don't want anyone watching me.

But more than that, I want these people to eat the delicious food I produce. And so, for decades now, I have cooked massive, complex meals in front of them all. And felt ashamed while doing so. And then I have served those meals and felt something like joy.

It seems I am willing to endure the exposure I fear in order to do something well.

The refrigerator again:
When my children were small, and I knew that they were worried or angry or scared but didn't want to talk about it, I would describe those emotions as being like food left in a refrigerator too long. "If you don't take out milk that's long past its due date, it starts to smell bad. That's what those emotions are like. You have to get them out of you or they sour."

I actually think that helped them at times.

The "gift of ADHD":
I absolutely despise that phrase.

ADHD hurt me too much throughout my childhood for me to see it as a gift—not without tagging on a lot of caveats. It may *contain* gifts. But that doesn't make it a gift. It makes it, at best, a kind of inside-out Trojan horse with some good stuff hidden away within the bad.

Or anyway, that's how it's been for me.

Yes, it is true that people with ADHD are often able to perceive connections between things that other people, more grounded in neurotypical thinking, may not grasp. People with ADHD are prone to *associative thinking*, which is of tremendous value if you want to do things like find metaphors in a kitchen appliance as a way to encourage your kids to tell you what has been worrying them.

And in that instance, ADHD also helps by giving you a working knowledge of what happens to food that's been lost for weeks in the back of the fridge.

So I guess that can be a gift. Of sorts.

It's never simple, is it?

Nothing is ever simple. But there are patterns in one's life that can help make even complicated phenomena come clear.

I love interior design. We have moved around a lot, and with each move, I throw myself into renovating, choosing perfect paint colors, reupholstering old furniture, hanging art artfully. I know very few people who get as much joy out of arranging a home as I do.

But then, without meaning to, I fill it with clutter. I make messes of my beautiful, harmonious spaces until they are all eventually versions of my childhood bedroom.

And those holiday meals? Each one is preceded by a few frantic days of cleaning—after which there is usually one room filled to the rafters with crap; crap that will explode back into my gorgeous spaces once everyone has left.

Because I will endure almost anything for even the fleeting, unfamiliar feeling of being able to do something well. And of being able to create beauty; because I grew up believing I could only create mess.

But—this is the important part—the feeling of shame always comes back. I may have created beauty, but the mess can only be pushed down for so long.

***The day I learned how other people label files*:**

I was talking to a friend about labeling drafts of stories so they can be readily found, and she mentioned that her computer files always have the date on them, or a number that denotes the order in which she wrote them.

A list of a few of the files on my computer:
JohnParkertheonewhereClaraeatsTuna
JohnParkertheonewhereClarashairisdescribedatlength
JohnParkerHappierEnding
JohnParker
ClaraNoJohnParkerBeforeIthoughtofhim
JPAugust
ClaraSpringwhenIhadthatreallybadcold

Something I have finally accepted, in my sixties:
I cannot do systems. They defeat me. Or maybe I defeat them.

Which approach to computer files is better?
Oh, I don't know. A part of me longs for order and envies the mind that thinks like that. But I do get tired of envying other people's minds. So I want to say there's something wrong with being so predictable and orderly, kind of sterile. Impersonal. Anyone can label things numerically. (Except me, I guess.) I *want* to say there's something wrong with being organized, but I suspect I'd be outvoted.

Still, sometimes, almost guiltily, I detect an appealing creativity to my own chaos, and I wonder if anyone who is organized ever envies me. Even as I curse myself for being unable to find the file I wrote in January 2006 (JohnParkerwhereHaroldisntinit).

Sometimes, I can *almost* see chaos as an advantage.

The gift of ADHD?
No comment.

What my advisor should have said:
"My own refrigerator is very well organized, which tells you something

about me. I'm tidy. Are we meant to learn something about this character from hers being somewhat chaotic?"

That's what he should have said. Because honestly, how can you teach fiction writing, if you think everyone does everything the same way?

But maybe that's just how neurotypical people think. Maybe they are so used to fitting in, that they never see beyond the "norm." Maybe they really are penned in by their abilities.

Though, to be fair, I did learn quite a bit from him at other times.

Something to keep in mind as you read this:
Human beings are complex, and complexity is sometimes another word for contradictory. We are none of us the characterological equivalent of rivers that flow in only one direction. We are more like multiple weather systems swirling every which way all at once.

I feared that if I was seen clearly, I would be deemed bad.

But I hated being misunderstood, so I wanted to be seen clearly.

I was sure that there was more to me than the sum total of the many tasks at which I was mysteriously inept. Even as I feared that there was not.

Yet more on the subject of refrigerators:
My daughter's high school boyfriend once cleaned out our refrigerator, unasked. Because he couldn't stand it.

Yet more on the subject of shame:
My daughter's high school boyfriend once cleaned out our refrigerator, unasked. Because he couldn't stand it.

On reading as self-medication:
There was no chaos when I read as a child. There were no physical objects I had to keep track of, nothing to be tidied, nothing to be found. There was just someone telling me a story and me understanding the story. Everything else disappeared.

On writing as self-medication:
There is no chaos when I write. There is no physical mess to sort through, no room to be tidied, nothing that I have lost that needs to be found. There is just me telling you a story, and working to find ways for it to convey what I cannot convey in any other form.

Everything else disappears.

Until the long periods when I just can't write.

My perennial advice to everyone suffering from "writer's block":
Every writer I know is someone who has felt that they were being silenced at some early, critical point in their life. They write because being silenced made them want to speak out. They write because being silenced is intolerable. They write because having tried to be silent, they are angry all the time. And the dam breaks.

But it isn't so easy to consistently overcome those silencing voices. Sometimes we can, but sometimes the voices win, and we stop writing for a bit—maybe for a long while. And when that happens, you have to get angry at being silenced, at any implication that you should be silent. You have to get angry at being shamed.

You have to reclaim your right to be heard. Even if you are scared to death of being seen.

The seesaw:
I am sitting on both ends, sometimes as a child, sometimes as an adult. On one end, there's the me who believes she is a failure as a human being, inherently bad. She is trying to make herself as inconspicuous as possible. And on the other end sits the me who as a child read in bed every night, and in doing so learned about the complexities of human beings and acquired an understanding of them that she didn't often detect in those around her; the me who discovered a way to calm the chaos in her head and in her surroundings, and who began using her outsider status to observe real people, not just the ones in books; the me who started to believe that maybe she had important

things to say, and that she had to risk exposure because it was the only way to be genuinely understood.

Sometimes one version of me is up; sometimes the other is. But I think that may be preferable to both of them hanging in midair, staring at one another, frozen in place.

The actual subject of the short story that has survived in my memory as "the one with the comment about refrigerator organization in the margin":
A young boy is trying to escape the chaos of his dysfunctional household by inventing a false identity for himself at a nearby neighbor's home.

Why I share these accounts of my shame:
To keep my emotional refrigerator clean.

Chapter 8 of My Life Story:
The woman who administered Robin's eventual ADHD evaluation was in her twenties and must have been good at a lot of things that Robin couldn't do, because she was a top resident at a very prestigious medical center. And she looked pulled together. Polished. As Robin took the tests (*she* was in her forties and looked a mess), it was clear that she was unable to accomplish a lot of the tasks in the given time. And this woman, accustomed to working with children, said something encouraging along the way. "Don't feel bad," she said. "This is meant to be challenging."

But . . .

But . . .

But . . .

But . . .

Robin couldn't quite find the words, but she *didn't* feel bad. Not at all. She felt relief. Yes, there was something unusual about her, just as she had guessed all along, but it wasn't a moral failing, not *laziness*, *slovenliness*, *grossness*, *disobedience*.

It was something neurological, just some atypical wiring. There's no shame in a thing like that. *Hallelujah!*

And all the ride home, she wept and wept.

And then, the next day, she went back to work, her mind a point of beautiful calm among the chaos and the clutter of her room.

PROMPT: The Thought Loosener

A collage essay, like the one above, is built around the kind of associative thinking and logic that comes naturally to many people who have ADHD. It skips around and tells a story out of order, with lots of asides. It can be very freeing to write in this manner, whether nonfiction or fiction. Here are some ideas to get you started. Try writing a collage essay or story using one or more of these as subject headings:

- My first thought when I hear the word ______:
- Why I am afraid of ______:
- The memory I am always trying to forget:
- Three habits in other people that I despise:
- Everything I know about my parents:
- Something that invariably makes me blush:

7

Train Rumbles by at 2:22 A.M., Every Monday Morning

ALLISON ADELLE HEDGE COKE

There's a narrowing angle when something definitive appears. A glance into spectacle, spectacular, delightful, distinct, significant, in otherwise mundane mist. In minutia, miracles freely optimizing space, spatial reason, defining rest, impression, embraced, adored, coalescence, Fibonacci configuration, what is meaning, most.

Each entry into *must* seizes *should* and alerts *instead* heightening ability to enact insight, hypervigilance, streaming awareness in sweeping luminous wave for precise enlightenment through some spectacle in wait for just a moment's notice, or the long-set-aside alternative musts, in stacks of unmet, just a day or so, dust-gathering city skylines arranged in cosmopolitan arrangements, books, papers, mail, to do, to do, to do, now draw succinct action, new arrangement, cleaning, here comes ninety-something quick set-asides to conquer, before drafting, then destroying, or losing the tenth draft, or so, until so many set-asides confuse targeting ideals, let alone sadness in leaving delicate insteads offering so much more—

Glistened point, shimmer, sunlight strike leaf vein pulse, resplendent, radiant, reach—everything, here, light through leaf, translucent glinting, momentary illumination, so much more than everything over there, split fissure focuses in splendor. This. World reels, winds up, narrowly shining lift to embetter something. If the day goes by and nothing completes what was worth it is refracting points in parallel embrace. Too many gorgeous inklings pass by in tasking flurries. Furious flinting hope leaves long lines leveraging angle to hold close sensory pleasure, stimulating open-wide beauty, blazing—

It'snotthistheywant

is it

Incessant beauty ignored for chores, for blight-out blanding in homogenized normality in fit-in within anticipated laters long after overdue and overdone.

All the while fifty-sixty others were completed in procrastination efforts a sway away from feat. Brainstorm lightnings strike through, peeling asphalt up from ground cover like twisters in the Southern Plains, or way ebbed flow from spouting tower funnels forming out in sea somewhere. Then begin again, unsettled with what was before, the scratches then, now myriad mix toward maybe this, all the while just wishing for the lighted leaf.

Slippery, this path. Mucky, muddy, musty, matters, in musts.

Much more perceptible, tangible, reasoned, left to one's own miracle mind fill.

Every single strand might meld anytime, all of it, maybe the thing. The curtain's furl on maple floor, that line of shadow from leaves on the other side of pane, ceiling fan neat, fridge hum, tinnitus, rattling somewhere, but the dog, too, unsettled, pacing, pacing until floor calls out and begs to be sprawled out on and she stretches so long and sighs, letting her legs run way after she's fallen out. Somewhere a world without wonder, but here it is everywhere all day through—until the lull, the flat-out, crash, binge, ennui, reel after reel fostering complete disquiet ignoring any feat possible, possibility, in exchange for drifting daydream, or shift away from present into other implications, artful, or not. In tunneling deeper, cove depth, stalagmite baseline, cool depth away from streaming rise, nothingness meditation, nevermore grave, behind, behind—brought by burden-musts, assigned tasking, outside idea-scape pestering festerous wound wound rapidly oppositional counterintuitive mal-wired maddening, mustering implausible condition so many movies might push far into abyss, where no one can forbid mighty acts, dream entanglement, where imperception of marveling may never maneuver over pristine acumen, what are we but banal when placed versus changing worlds.

In the stillness, wall shadows, shaking leaves, can the world be rid of me yet. Might something occur where one can vanish imperceptible erased.

This night-blooming cereus, most incredible scent, complex construction, mesmerizing princess of the night, slow-simmered soup for Cantonese, bees begin accumulating pollen, moving one leg, the other, early light just as the flower begins its fold for day, closure into slumbering time, loosely letting petals join so to say what is here is only divined in dark, in light of the moon, or reflective time. Consider "Jade Steps Grieving" and the night princess wandering down in wait, maybe two seasons from here, stockings gauzed, the moon still the moon, sometimes we drink with it, too, especially when flowers bloom, like here, now, these night-blooming cereus, so brilliantly wavering minds who meet them, companions, comrades, or lovers lost in luminous glow. Li Bai maintains memory while Wang Wei's cold plum flowers somewhere along a windowsill in the village of the mind's eye. The wilt here brings morning, still the scent intoxicates.

Once, some kid in my youth played Russian roulette in Raleigh. Only once. Shot still follows most of us he knew. Another whose eye went out way further than my lazy one, noted it glass from another shot a friend playing around kicked off. Or the arm my sister broke when my brother tried to block the door, so she'd stay home like we had to, with all the noise of madness there. The neighbor kid losing their uncle under train trestle to concrete when he didn't see the light. Or the baby skunk so like a kitten Dad had me release. All those early reckonings, alongside instruments making music manifest, or records spinning storied lives.

Crickets flail legs to flute temperature readings in warmer winds than this. La Niña is still here. El Niño missed us this atmospheric rivering, proxy for forecasts, traditionally wet or dry, no more. Chaotic convergence, climate-shifting currents, any way the wind blows, *doesn't really matter. Mama*. Storms killed twelve this month.

A total eclipse coming nigh about a week before the Lyrids. A point in the night sky is radiant. Quadrantids just left a bit ago. Some fireballs may be plausible.

Neighing horses near me bring me peace. Besties. Remember the night we caught the lunar eclipse out riding with the starshine.

Furniture mirrors on maple floor from overhead light. Looks a bit noir right now. Like a street in rain with traffic and neon lights shining on the wet, wet world. Good to have a dry house when so many others are without. It's why we share space, to fully enjoy.

Maybe you're all about light and dark, wet, and dry. The freezer should have some frozen bananas, dairy-free ice cream, but the water isn't working on the door of it. Someone pushed too hard when the ice was blocking flow, and now it just shoots out ice and no water comes at all. In about an hour we might see a shooting star, wait, no that was then.

Everyonceinawhile the sky is right, unfolding possible, release, most proficient results occur. It's the pinnacle. Maybe you read that book. A few have. Someone is speaking on it at work this week. Funny thing is, it was written in her home when she wasn't there. In a weekend of blissful open-wide flowing, furious let-go, unfolding, unfurling, succinct daydreaming flow. Deadline was mine.

Theirs too, didn't matter, nothing really matters.

Until the next time, this what is what and more of this and that. Fidgeting is the way of the world, until the wonder unravels—

On jury duty, each lunch break, ate at M's, watched *Jury Duty* on iPhone, returned to court noticing only two of us moved constantly during long questioning of potential jurists. Only two of us. So obvious the parallel beat. Percussive in the droning debate of could you, would you, what have you, or were you in your deepest fright. No matter, so heinous, all was wanted was escape. Came late, down to last nine when the final were selected and we, relieved.

The ice cream is melting now, rice bowls we got at the dog rescue thrift store will salvage some.

Is it raining yet?

Get into place, position, and the rest will follow. Isn't that the way of this world. Move toward what must be done and be done with it. In the meantime, mellowing when allowed, when give oneself permission to let go, cast out, flow, and find the acumen available if we just attend to it. Unfold, let the mind meld onto the page so that static evacuates as if under mandatory order. Such a relief, such a break in the everyday when it is allowed, allowable. Maybe a retreat—

Some student submissions just came through. Due two nights ago. It's ok, I'm pretending not to notice, not to be aware of everything.

Maybe flee, move, have a life somewhere poetry is quietly profound. Firecrackers blaring night sky, or stillness in moonlight along luminescent shoreline when bioluminescent plankton visit blueing the world with shimmering glow. For now, it's applications to grad school, so many gorgeous glimmers of potential, maybe genius for all of us to foster, carefully, like curating espresso to find its full flavor, *Luminous Method*, like Sze, Levertov, Miles. Josephine Miles, though Miles Davis did, too, bring out the best of every player made, including Herbie Hancock, who played a wrong note, really wrong note, and Miles took a beat, played in return making it the exact right note to play, changing worlds with intentionality rarely rivaled. *One more cup of coffee for the road—*

Better make this pour decaf, eventually will have to rest. One eye open to get everything due done, way past time, but tonight is prime, so the time it should actually happen. Original deadline had no call, no matter of more, just matter of fact. Never happens. Now is now. Being *in time*, now, here, with it.

The dog next to me sleeps with one eye open, as well. Raises her head now and then, looks, sighs, rests, running from time to time, in place on her left side. Right now both sets of paired legs are easily crossed and her breathing makes me think of music.

Ramón Palomares had a wonderful poem about a dog running through the camp. Like me he came from fields. Sometimes they're with me still. Maybe all the time, really. Do you ever fully leave the fields when you came of age in them? Maybe so. Maybe the field's furrows fill your brow when you age, grow old. Maybe they are the strokes of keyboard and along the tray fingers find furrows between the keyed rows.

Isn't it all so beautiful, this world. So many things to consider, to rest upon, be with. When something conditions you, grab it and hold on, it's time, now. Stay with it as long as it leads you, that's when the read that's necessary comes to be.

8

Divergence as Praxis, the Accretion of Force, and Feeling Professional

Working Through Grief, Pain, Recovery, Setbacks, and—

KHADIJAH QUEEN

This piece, in an earlier form, was delivered on January 5, 2024, at the 2024 MLA Convention in Philadelphia.

SETTING: [Describe conference room. The seating is _____. The lighting is _____. The exits are _____.] Constant low sound plays in background (and each set of dots on the page henceforth is a breath; sometimes with optional space around it) to mimic the unmedi(c)ated interior:

> ACCRETION OF FORCE
> ..
> ..
> YES

Speaker (visual description):

> Khadijah Queen, a brown-skinned Black woman with curly salt-and-pepper hair that falls to her shoulders. She has brown eyes

and red lipstick. She is wearing an off-white cashmere turtleneck, black midi skirt, and black suede pointed-toe boots. She is wearing gold and silver hoop earrings, a beaded bracelet with lava rock and malachite, and a silver Apple Watch. She has ADHD and does not make eye contact with the audience so that she is free to hyperfocus on the text in front of her.

Text to be read aloud (Speaker has provided sections to volunteer readers in the audience):
What is incapable of softening. A stance. A material. A belief. A religion. An institution.

..

We are told.
We learn to believe.
We agree to authority.

(What comes first, in this agreement? Care or force? Which [is] matter[s]—?)

We surrender to consequence—its threats, its realities.
For our own good. Our own (really?) protection.
Our acceptance into.
We participate. (One kind of sustaining.)

We also feel.
What we feel and what we are told to feel, or told we *should* feel, often fail
to match. We learn to perceive

duty as honor. Sacrifice as toughness. Stoicism, silence—admirable. Long hours in suits and libraries and offices fail to qualify as visual toil—intellectual feeling seen/perceived in material comfort, in rarefied air. We practice physical packaging of interior denials. We agree in public to ignore what we feel in the interior—tired, afraid, hungry, in need or want of care or rest; pained, grieving, bullied, forced—and we appear.

..

So as not to appear—or be perceived—as in need, or childlike, the only states of approved yet inconvenient, pitiable or despised public vulnerability. So as to pretend to reify the false veneer.

..

We appear with our expertise—dare we mention the term *special interest*—and not (we say)(or pretend to believe)(or shape into acceptable expression) the feeling that first led us to the Subject(s) in which we have become expert, our interest led by quick brains, dopaminic pathways toward the self in approved fashion. Our feelings of rebellion transformed into intellectual modes of acceptance. Our resistances, made academic, morphed into service pathways, methods of exchange, leading to (sometimes) feelings of diminishment—grandiosity of extremes turned realistic, feeling like a cup of salt held in a closed mouth.

Resistance is a hard feeling. I encounter resistance within myself when confronted with externalized force.

..

What place does such feeling have in an institution? Are the two incompatible? Can we consider, as in a poem, holding apparently opposing or contradictory things in the same (physical/language) space? Can we allow for their coexistence? Can we allow for adjustments to collective belief?

..

In 2016, I wrote in a poem:

> "My mother is familiar with duty & made me so / I can't live on that loss."

I was speaking about family, alive and dead, here in form and felt in spirit. Unhinging from my father—a conman, forever demanding a daughter's duty, but rarely delivering a father's. I learned to understand duty as care by force, and care by choice as love.

..

What is the role of love in professional contexts? Who defines love in public? Do we publicly understand love as care by choice, unromantic?

Is a feeling soft, or hard? If the latter, what happens when/if it softens?

..

I was speaking about authority. The unnamed policeman
who killed my brother in 1977 & made me so
I could not know him past infancy except as a ghost.

..

If I say grief is a wave, infinite and undulant, what do you feel?

Does what you feel resemble resistance, or relief? What about when another person who looks like your dead brother is killed on television, ad infinitum, recorded on the interior of public minds, externalized, electronic ghosts imagined out of their bodies, their last feelings pained into physical absence?

..

What if you are "at work" having such soft, uncontainable feelings? Is your work/life in balance? What is the fulcrum of such balance? What does it feel like—inside? How does that inside feeling translate into action that soothes or suppresses what you feel? How does it feel to believe that how you feel doesn't matter outside of you? Does your feeling affect your performance? Do you have to apologize for the externalization of your interior reality as physically manifested feeling, if your brain cannot control the drowning wave of feeling, that unsupported and inconvenient sadness?

..

Wind-based divergence in water bodies creates an upwelling, and depresses the surface. What lies below rises, and spreads beneath the waves, undeniable, disruptive. An energy shift. An interruption of flow.

Some things need to be disrupted—

> *At least six people in unison imitate the wind, in sounds and/or movement*

..

Muriel Rukeyser said: "The work that a poem does is a transfer of human energy." Before she was blacklisted, during the McCarthy era, she wrote that the imagination connected poetry and the sciences. An equation of the impossible: the deployment of theory and practice as feeling in the body, as emotion, as animating

consciousness simultaneously, delivered through language—mediated by or contained in page or voice, then transferred to the reader, the perceiver.

Do you have the energy? At work

what feeling is transferred in teaching? In research? In committee meetings?
In an email, starting

> *At least three other voices in unison*: [I hope this finds you]

..

..

..

..

Speaker sits or stands, but is silent. A recording plays:

> If I record myself reading this personal professional paper and play the recording in conference space instead of using my living voice, if instead of performing I watch only the audience perform a real or performed reaction to the recorded performance, what will be different in terms of feeling?

Speaker resumes:
Certain disabilities create an abundance of feeling.
And, an awareness of many feelings at once.
One could also call such abundance chaos.
How to choose one word or the other, as a state. Feeling or not-feeling,
reconciling feeling and belief, abundant mind externalized in a restricted public body. Trying to decide on institution—a living process.

..

..

If I feel, I must force.
My way into not-feeling, the institution says. (A container, for the uncontainable.)

If I feel light. If I feel sound. If I feel smell.

A field, an endless horizon.

> *Another voice*: One you cannot reach the end of.

..

..

A recording plays:

> A loss is a destabilizing force. Death changes the living left. If that death comes from collective cultural inaction (CCI—yes I made it an official term by giving it an acronym), grief morphs into moral injury. If two deaths come from CCI, deaths of two mother-elders who share my blood invaded by a deadly public virus, if disability comes from CCI, countless denials of its significance, well—the anger comes. If millions die from CCI—
>
> ..
>
> Who knows what the body does to process such power without release?
> A force throughout the body, the unprotected
> outside, attacking its mirror-soft interior.
>
> ..

I try to soften my resistance to being
hardened
pleasantly, capably present
in hostile environments.

Speaker resumes (or passes around as a side note, a diversion of related thought, functioning as the unsaid, or unacceptable belief): The grocery store parking lot, with Trump trucks and armed Southern men. The doctor's office, where I must prove my invisible pain exists even when tests affirm—the everlasting fight for care. And yes, I try to soften my resistance to work. Not work as in teaching or writing, which I love to the point of hyperfocus, but work as in maintaining the institutional illusion of emotionless busyness

unless that emotion is blandly pleasant. A shell of smiles in feigned or forced efficiency. The meetings in which my imagination (what got me employed) will not get deployed. Trapped, in bureaucratic gravel I cannot translate into anything I can discern as logical or efficient—another definition of work.

Work, where imagination terrifies existing institutional practice, and therefore meets resistance. Work, where I feel and see my colleagues' horror at my out-loud, off-paper divergent thought, yet they polish the smooth shell of kindness in words. In the shining reflection of such steel constructions, I feel the pressure to lessen myself into some mysterious common baseline I am not capable of comprehending.

I refuse to call it a mask.

In my shell I am busy filling out forms
answering emails
adjusting pleasantly to changes in processes
and fail.

..

..

My young adult son calls neurotypical people *neurobasic*. I was born in 1975. The year American troops left Saigon and Franco died. The Khmer Rouge came into power and so did Margaret Thatcher. Someone(s) tried to kill Gerald Ford, twice. I am a Gemini. My hyperactivity is interior; my impulsivity is not. Late in life, I learned about my Leo: moon, rising, Venus. I love a good list. Some institutional names for *attention-deficit hyperactivity disorder* before 1980:

- Abnormal defect of moral control
- Organic Brain Disease
- Disease of attention
- Minimal brain damage
- Minimal brain dysfunction
- Minimal brain disorder
- Hyperkinesis
- Hyperkinetic Reaction of Childhood
- Hypermetamorphosis
- Hyperactive child syndrome
- Unstable nervous system
- Clumsy Child Syndrome [I lose count of the bruised decades]

These days some of us like to joke about our executive dysfunction. I have an Etsy sticker somewhere: *Well, well, well, if it isn't the consequences of my own . . .*

On TikTok, I cozy up to the term *neurospicy*. I like the sound. I like the flavor.

..

My psychiatrist refills my stimulant medication. I do not respond well to SSRIs because ____ (a suspicion). I joke that I am not depressed, that my brain just needs a little help to make more dopamine. He tells me there is no such thing as dopamine deficiency. I don't argue because my logical mind tells me that would fail to make efficient use of my [not unlimited] energy. Ha. Ha.

..

Speaker resumes:
I try to soften my resistance to being.

..

In 2011, I wrote in a poem: "I want my softness to be safe."

The texture of want
can be hard; an accretion of force.

Speaker sits, is silent.

Another voice: If a feeling is allowed to accumulate without release, the accretion of feeling is overwhelm.

Another voice: Sometimes, you can feel overwhelm before it overtakes.

Another voice (in a whisper): Does the institution overwhelm? In its parts or as a whole? In theory or in practice?

Another voice: A simile: overwhelm like a wave. A metaphor: waves of stimuli can drown you.

..

A recording plays (or Speaker passes around as a side note, or a bibliography and a set of follow-up questions):

In 2022, Dr. Bettina Judd distinguished *feeling* from *feelin*: "feelin, in African American Vernacular English," she writes, "is how Black women artists approach and produce knowledge as internal and complex, entangled with pleasure, pain, anger, and joy, and manifesting artistic production itself as the meaning of the work."

Does being a Black woman in America separate me from everyone else?
Does the truncation of origins separate me from everyone else?
Does my refusal to participate in gaslighting separate me from everyone else?

Said another way:

> *Another voice*: Am I (or will I ever be) considered part of anyone's *all*, really?
> *Another voice*: Am I (or will I ever be) considered, really?
> *Another voice*: How does that information feel to know, or believe, or resist?

..

A recording plays, and the Speaker may or may not read along, aloud:

If I say I feel wholly unconsidered in most American settings, institutional or otherwise, would you believe that feeling, or try to convince me that what I feel isn't real?

Whose beliefs matter most? What if some hardened beliefs are ghosts of the unloved, the shell of duty masking the literal and physical feeling of want of care?

If I say I feel I have lived through infinite accretions of force, can you imagine what that feels like? Or do you (let yourself) feel it, too?

Since we have all—at one point or another, if not now, still, and if not, let's pretend—agreed to work through the accretion of force, couldn't we all agree otherwise?

If we agree to practices that build wellness, and we create structures and systems that enable us to enact such practices, instead of creating hollow facades in electronic language that give appearance without reality—the word-ghosts of care—what would that feel like?

In my imagination, that would feel like release.

Could that release start to soften hard institutional edges, dulling the sharpest points, the bruising rigidity, so that softness becomes a new and respected form of prestige?

Said another way:

> *Another voice*: What if welcoming and inclusion—in practice, not theory—became signs of prestige?
> *Another voice*: An accretion of thought becomes belief.

Speaker resumes (or passes around as a side note, a diversion in the form of constantly imagined escape into the appearance and feeling of safety in other colonizer countries):
When I spent time in France, and somewhat in Italy, I could walk in public. I could walk safely alone. I could exist outside without fear. I could eat without getting sick—the food wasn't poisoning me because the people created laws to protect themselves from damaging chemicals American agribusiness chooses for profit. The people chose to protect themselves instead of an institution. (They chose the soft institution of food.) I could walk in nature without thinking about lynchings—in general, and of my great-grandfather specifically: John White, of Autaugaville, Alabama, a hundred years ago, hard evidence of which I could only find in the haunted tone of the story passed

down, and the town's haunted location between Selma and Montgomery. I could walk outside with my grown son and not think ghost-thoughts about the police and my brother Steven, or other Black people shot or fought or hung or dragged by other angry or hate-filled men in Trump trucks or hats or public uniforms or otherwise—a threat in general, and specifically, to make feeling and a body disappear in public, transferred as the energy of grief to the soft interiors of loved ones' DNA. An accretion of theory, as if by force:

..

A recording plays (what the Speaker does will be unpredictable, but probably not exciting):

> After a time, with care, by choice of feeling, allowance, imagination, belief—grief softens. Anger softens. I soften. I feel more like my real self, and not the hard shell I've learned I must force myself to maintain, or risk harm in the institution, even though the shell itself is harm, and the soft interior becomes the escape, however contained the physical appearance in public, ever uncontainable when protected, loved, however secret, or perceived as ghost.
>
> And the unyielding yields.
>
> And the softness provides comfort.
>
> And the presence of force becomes irrelevant.

PROMPT: Unyielding Spaces

Write a poem, scene, essay, or story about a place that withholds something from its inhabitants. The thing withheld can be knowledge, sustenance, joy, or even *un*happiness. This place can be real or imagined. Include someone or something who/that tracks what is unsaid. Where does that mystery reside? What is the cost of its withholding? Use a color and a natural element as two central themes.

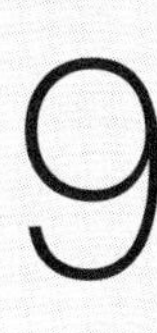

The End Game

On Struggle, Style, Syntax, and Sustainability

JAMI NAKAMURA LIN

part one: struggle

1. When I was eighteen, I printed out a quote and taped it to my bedroom wall: "I can't go on, I must go on, I'll go on." It was by Samuel Beckett. By then I'd been hospitalized several times. I'd just been diagnosed with bipolar I. I tried to make it to the end of each day, which often felt insurmountable.
2. I often believe I will never be able to reach the end of anything: only stuck forever, doggy-paddling.
3. Yet I have quite large aspirations. From the time I was a child, I spoke about the books I would publish in the future. I always knew this was what I wanted.
4. So on the one hand, I always knew I would write a book. On the other hand, I always knew I could never finish a book. Even after getting an agent, after the auction, after signing my book contract, I still did not believe I could do it. I had sold my memoir on proposal, which meant it mostly existed in my head. Many things that exist in my head never leave it. I told my therapist: I'm afraid the stress of writing this book will send me to the hospital again. I was kind of joking, but mostly not. A decade prior, the stress of graduate school had undone me, fraying my mind bit by bit until I ended

up in a psychiatric facility. Since then I had tried to keep my life as low stress as possible. But a book deadline meant stress. Especially a book like mine, which was about not only my bipolar but also my father's death.

5. In my book proposal, I wrote that I would turn in my first draft in six months. There was no need to give myself such a short time frame. No one was asking for this. I just thought that there was a better chance of selling it if they knew I could write it quickly. I have always had a hard time knowing my capacity. I overpromise. I want to make people happy, and in the end, I disappoint them. It's hard for me to be realistic.
6. But: what does *realistic* even mean? I do not know. I have never perceived things the way other people seem to perceive them. This misalignment has happened in a broad spectrum of ways. At one end, there are the bipolar hallucinations I experienced during one episode when I was seventeen. In the middle, there is the rejection sensitive dysphoria common in people with ADHD. And at the other end, the most frequent end, there is the fact that the things I focus on are often different than what other people focus on. We can be watching the same movie, but our eyes are zoomed in on such different aspects that it looks like two different films entirely.
7. At the time I sold my book, I did not know I had ADHD. I had suspicions, inklings, but I was used to connecting everything—my quirks, my needs, my ailments—to my bipolar, as doctors had done since I was diagnosed. I was used to ignoring things. But after turning in my first draft to my editor—after a two-week extension, which I am happy to say I learned to ask for ahead of time—I got a neuropsychiatric evaluation and a diagnosis.
8. When researching my new diagnosis, I found that when it comes to ADHD and writing, many of the so-called strategies are centered around *process*—how we organize our schedules and our lives to support the way our minds work. How to be productive. How to channel hyperfocus. How to overcome distraction.

9. This is, of course, important. Learning what time of day my brain was sharpest was key (9–11 a.m. and 9–11 p.m.—untraditional, but it works for me). I learned that if I don't see something, it basically doesn't exist, so I do most of my drafting and research in longhand. (Plus, a blank page intimidates me less than a blank computer screen.) When I'm researching or note-taking, I use a system of full-stick Post-it notes and an enormous journal with a double-page spread for each topic. It's like having a lot of different corkboards in one spot.
10. But what I am more interested in is how our neurodivergence affects the *style* of our writing. What little information about ADHD and writing style I could find was often like the kind I found in an article in an ADHD magazine, which says that the difficulty with writing for ADHD students is not in idea formation, but in transferring ideas onto the page. Because ADHD writers write with less detail, the article states: "Encourage colorful description. Students with ADHD often have difficulty 'dressing up' their written words. Help them add adjectives and use stronger, more active verbs in sentences."[1]
11. But what if we don't *want* our writing to hide our neurodiverse thinking? There are limited studies that show that ADHD children have distinctive linguistic patterns. I want to parse our writing, our natural styles, and see its patterns, rhythms, textures. I want to let that be the beating heart of our writing, not something to be excised.
12. I do not know much about this field of research, but I do know that the only way I was able to finish *The Night Parade* was by having the work mimic my own style of thinking, one that is fragmented, circular, associative, and not tethered to time and space in the usual way.

1 Chris A. Zeigler Dendy, "How to Remove Hurdles to Writing for Students with ADHD," *ADDitude*, September 7, 2022, www.additudemag.com/write-well/.

13. Many of my interviews when the book came out went something like this:

> **Interviewer:** Why, in your book, did you choose to incorporate so much white space? Were you influenced by the groundbreaking work of X and Y, who also use discrete text blocks with large margins?
>
> > No—it's because it's hard for me to read a long paragraph. It's hard for me to focus when there are so many words in one block. I formatted the book in a way that would be easy for me to read.
>
> **Interviewer:** You don't use quotation marks for dialogue. Often, writers put such dialogue in italics. Why did you decide not to use italics?
>
> > Because it's hard for me to read italics.
>
> **Interviewer:** Your work is so innovative, using so many different points of view and perspectives. I particularly love Chapter X, which does Y. How did you decide to do that?
>
> > It didn't feel so much like a choice, but the only option after months spent bashing my head against the wall, trying to write it any other way.

14. I tried to write the book in what I thought of as the "regular way." And I could not. Draft after draft of wringing my hands. If it had been easier for me to write this memoir in a more straightforward manner, perhaps I would have done it. But I couldn't. The writing flowed when I let it go the way my mind wanted. The book I ended up with was spiraling, shifting, speculative, moving all over in time and place, changing tenses and points of view, going through portals and wormholes and out again. A book that reflects how I think and how I feel and how I see. It came out this way because I could not do it the other way. The syntax, the structure, the style—all of these were choices I made because I had to, because I was on my fifth draft of a chapter and it was still wrong until I broke it open. Thankfully, my editor was very supportive. At one point she told me when I struggled, again, to relay a straightforward scene, marching forward in time: "Reality isn't your strong suit. Lean into the weird."

15. It would have been much easier if I had allowed myself to do this from the beginning. But I didn't know. We are trained to write as if we are all neurotypical. We are not often asked questions like: *How do you think? How can your writing reflect the unique ways you think?* Instead I had years of my MFA instructors telling me I couldn't do X or Y. They told me I needed scene, that I couldn't have so much exposition, that I couldn't tell my stories from so many different points in time.

16. But I love writing that lives on the periphery, on the borderlands. I believe neurodivergent writers are uniquely equipped to write from that place, with its friction and energy. Our brains literally find their own paths. This is difficult. And yet we do it.

17. So: I finished the book, an illustrated speculative memoir (a genre that, among other things, can embrace the fantastical to more fully realize the truth) that used yōkai and other Japanese, Taiwanese, and Okinawan monsters and spirits of legend to ask how we learn to live with the things that haunt us. Originally it was about my bipolar and my father's death, but it was writing itself that haunted me. The book's central concern became the difficulty of telling my story, of reckoning with an archive, and of shaping a narrative. That was the only way I could finish my book: by writing the anguish of creation into the created object itself.

18. And yet: one of the main reasons I was able to finish the book was that I was able to quit my day job, which was made possible by my book advance and having access to my husband's health insurance. My low energy means that if I had to keep working at the same time, it would have taken me so much longer—had I finished at all. (I think often of all the books missing from our bookshelves, the books not getting written, because of all the financial and structural barriers for neurodivergent, chronically ill, and disabled folks.) I finished it. I still feel unsure about being able to finish the second book, but I finished this one.

part two: syntax, style, structure

19. As I write this essay, it is November, and *The Night Parade* came out three weeks ago. Despite the anxiety of having my writing out in the world, I love that the book mirrors the way my mind works. So many of the syntactical, stylistic, and structural choices I made were a direct result of specific struggles I encountered while writing.

20. For example: notice how the sentences in this essay are all short, abrupt, subject-verb-object. This is because I am struggling to write it. When I have a hard time, I let my sentences be simple. I sometimes feel embarrassed about this. Like: *Oh, readers will think I am not a good writer, because my sentences are not complex and beautiful.* I am trying to extricate these thoughts. If it helps me write, this is what I should do. I learned this, again, through trial and error. One of the earliest essays I wrote that was then adapted into *The Night Parade* was about my miscarriage. I hadn't written anything in months. I felt so stalled, until I let myself dispense with my normal, more lyrical writing and just write in these choppy chunks. You can often tell what kind of mental state I'm in when drafting because the syntax of the sentences reflects it. (However, as I revise my drafts over and over again, this can change.)

21. For example: see how this essay is numbered like a list. Much of my writing is organized like this. My brain feels all over the place, so giving myself a structure, even the false momentum of ascending numbers, can give it the order I need.

22. For example: in my book, I dispensed with everything that was hard for me to read. I always skim over physical description. My brain cannot grasp it. I have very little spatial reasoning or sense of geography—I am always covered in bruises, unsure where my body is in relation to the door or the table. When I read, I cannot imagine what is being described, so I have skipped those parts since I was a child. In my own book, I just didn't put any in. The emotional landscape is well described, but the physical? Almost invisible. I think we often are taught we *must* include certain things, and I do not think this is true.

23. For example: I prefer things that move quickly, both in my books and outside of them. Speed provides the dopamine I crave. I like works like *One Hundred Years of Solitude*, which have a kind of narrative speed, often moving through vast swaths of time quickly. I tried for so long to write scenes with action that unfolds. And then I thought: What if I just didn't? I don't mean to say that I love fast-paced action—most of my favorite things have no action. I just prefer telling to showing. Summary gets a bad rap, but often I think the problem is not exposition or summary but rather that we write these in a way that is not animated, that is not interesting, that is merely an info dump.

24. For example: structurally, I can't keep track of more than a chapter's worth of information, so each chapter in my memoir is self-contained, like an essay. When I was writing each chapter, I didn't have to think about the material in the other chapters. I am writing my next book, a novel, in the same way—after, of course, writing 50,000 words I got lost in. I just can't hold on to that much information. I started writing that misguided draft because I thought that's how *real* novels were written, instead of asking myself what would allow *me* to finish my novel, or even remembering what helped me finish my first book. (I worked so hard to figure out how to finish that first time, but then immediately forgot these tips and tricks. I had to figure them out again from scratch. I hope this time it will stick.)

part three: con/summation

25. It turns out I got the quote on my bedroom wall slightly wrong. The last line of Beckett's *The Unnamable* is ". . . before the door that opens on my story, that would surprise me, if it opens, it will be I, it will be the silence, where I am, I don't know, I'll never know, in the silence you don't know, you must go on, I can't go on, I'll go on."

26. I started a version of *this* essay in the car. Or rather, I spoke it out loud in the car, into my phone on my lap. The sounds of Chicago's 94 expressway—construction, zooming trucks—will clutter up the recording. It is not ideal. But this is also what will allow me to write it. Over the years, I've discovered techniques that make it easier to begin: being in certain locations, speaking instead of writing or typing. I've had to adapt to my needs. Now, finding the door that opens on my story is the easy part for me.

27. Finding the door that will lead me out is the hard part.

28. Right now I am finishing the essay in a coffee shop. It is due tomorrow. I usually don't write in coffee shops, but last night I had a little episode—more intense than I've had in months—because of accumulated stress, anxiety, seasonal depression, and grief at the current state of the world. The episode was triggered by grotesque images of mutilated fish that I'd seen when looking up our pet fish's illness. When I got stressed, these intrusive images started cascading in my mind, and my body started to agitate the way it used to in my bad bipolar episodes. I cried to my husband, dug under my weighted blanket, took a little bit of Xanax, and watched a reality show until I calmed down.

29. Today, as I parked my car in our driveway after dropping my daughter off at preschool, the intrusive images came back. My body flooded with adrenaline again. I wanted to watch the reality show again to distract myself, but this essay is due tomorrow.

30. Like many people with ADHD, I have a complicated history with deadlines. Without deadlines, it's hard for me to find the motivation to complete things. (My agent found *me* and encouraged me to create my book proposal, or else I probably wouldn't have put together the book for another few years, at least.) In graduate school, I was once hospitalized the day a huge project was due, one I'd procrastinated on and couldn't complete. More than a decade later, I still frequently work up to the last hour, but now I almost always finish, or I ask for an extension. I try to do a lot of the prep work beforehand.

31. So I knew I had to work on this essay today. My sister helped me with the plan: I would go inside the house. I would get the laptop. I would not look at the fish. I would drive to a coffee shop and listen to music very loudly on my headphones to block out the world and hopefully the intrusive thoughts.

32. So that is what I am doing. Do I wish this essay was different? Yes. Do I wish I had more time? Yes. This is how I feel about much of my writing, and yet I've had to learn to turn things in instead of waiting for perfection. I still am often flooded with embarrassment and shame when I turn such things in—these vestiges of the perfectionism that plagued me for so long. But I'm working on it. And I'm turning my writing in anyway. None of the editors did what I feared: Say it was terrible. Say I was an embarrassment.

33. In my head, I often framed this as lowering my standards. (And, when things were bad: lowering them even further, because otherwise I could not finish.) I am trying to reframe this as: realigning my standards to match up with my current capacity. Because while it's true that I often have unattainable ideals, it's also true that a lot of the time, my pieces *could* have reached them if I had more time or energy. Sometimes I do have that time and energy. Sometimes I don't. I am trying to hold both of these ideas at once, and realize that some pieces are not going to be as "good" as others, and that can be okay.

part four: sustainability

34. A 1996 *New York Times* review called Beckett's later work "demanding," unfriendly to the reader, unapproachable. On the one hand, I get it. I, too, struggled to read his work; I have no connection to his writing other than that line which has followed me through my life. (I'm a scavenger, picking out lines, scraps, using them as themes and structures later on. Sometimes I feel like everything I write is built on a house of cards.)

35. On the other hand, I empathize with his narrative position, what the reviewer David Gates called "a Ping-Pong volley of assertion and denial." To constantly be creatively cycling, rarely in equilibrium. We feel like it will be impossible to complete something. And it's true: sometimes we will not be able to finish, for whatever reason. But not completing something once does not mean we cannot finish anything ever.

36. I do not think I can finish my second book. I do not think I will get to the end. And yet I did for the first. I do. I will. I'll say the words again:

37. I don't know.
I'll never know.
In the silence you don't know.
You must go on.
I can't go on.
I'll go on.

PROMPT: A Page of One's Own

In this exercise, you'll identify styles, patterns, and aesthetics that you are drawn to in your daily life and then use them to figure out what writing processes and stylistic choices feel most natural to you. This will take about an hour to complete.

Part 1: Make Three Lists

Draw a vertical line down the middle of three sheets of paper. Write "Side A" on one side of each page and "Side B" on the other.

List 1: Your Ideal Space

Side A: Think about a space in which you feel calm and supported. List its attributes. (For example, "tidy and spacious.")

Side B: Look at each positive attribute you identified on Side A. List its opposite. (For example, the opposite of "tidy and spacious" might be "cluttered and cramped.")

Characteristics to consider: level of noise, temperature, color, light, aesthetics, spaciousness vs. crowdedness, urban vs. rural setting, natural vs. built environment

List 2: How You Interact with Stories

Side A: Think about what helps you engage with a story. List those attributes. (For example, "narrative speed.")

Side B: Think about what bores you or makes a story hard to follow. List those attributes. (For example, "scenic detail.")

Questions to consider: Do you prefer listening to audiobooks, physically turning the pages of a book, or watching TV? When do you tune in, tune out, skim, skip, or reread? Do you pause to ask questions, look things up, or write in the margins? What kinds of books did you enjoy as a kid?

List 3: Translate Your Preferences

Side A: Look at the positive attributes you listed on side A of both lists. Translate each attribute into a writing style, pattern, or aesthetic. (For example, "tidy and spacious" might translate to "simple sentences and wide margins.")

Side B: Look at the negative attributes you listed on side B of both lists. Translate each attribute into a writing style, pattern, or aesthetic. (For example, "interruptions" might translate to "fragmented or braided narratives.")

Part 2: Li(s)tmus Test

Think of a simple story that you know well (for example, a fairy tale, the plot of a children's movie, or a family anecdote). Write "Story A" on one sheet of paper and "Story B" on another.

Story A: Write the story using the positive attributes you identified on side A of list 3 ("Translate Your Preferences").

Story B: Write the story using the negative attributes you identified on side B of list 3 ("Translate Your Preferences").

Part 3: Figure Out Your Writing Style

Compare the two stories you wrote in part 2, and answer the following questions:

- Which story flowed more easily?
- How did you feel in your body while writing each one? (For example, "calm and centered.")
- What was your thought process like during each one? (For example, "I got distracted toward the end.")
- Were there negative traits that you actually enjoyed?
- Were there positive traits that didn't engage you?

Your answers to these questions will help guide you toward a writing style that supports the unique way your mind works.

10

Ghosts by the Light of My ADHD

LAWRENCE-MINH BÙI DAVIS

I'm going to start right here in a swell of what I experience as release:

thought and sensation, oh, and memory, beginning to drain from what feels
like a basin
of waking lucidity, down a whole miniature network of channels
like tiny glowy cilia to somewhere
far below,

you are near, I think. They
and— haven't found each other yet. I can
feel the distance between
them;

they're close but still so far
apart. I'm not sure they even know
each other yet. They . . . hurt. I think. . . . I think
my father is drowning. No, not that kind of
drowning. The other kind. He needs her, my

mother. He doesn't know it yet, but
he needs h

Not sure what the
rest of that sentence was

going to be before it was, ah, cut short.
I remember wanting to say something about the stilled surface of being alive.

The passage above and to the right is the cacophony of being dead. It's a message from a ghost. I don't know where it came from. It just interrupted, as ghosts sometimes do.

I'm in the late stages of writing a novel, titled *GHOST ƠI*, about ghosts and the spirit mediums through whom ghosts sometimes speak, or put another way, incarnate. Of the many names for the many kinds of spirit mediums, my favorite is probably thế của bổn phu, which translates from the Vietnamese to something like "seat for the spirits." I'm also fond of người có đồng, sometimes translated as "person having the fate of a medium." I'm not a person having the fate of a medium, but I am a person having the fate of trying to write about a person having the fate of a medium, and maybe what the fates of mediums broadly, in our late capitalist world, have to tell us.

My impulse was to open this essay by grounding myself in listening, to myself, in the moment of starting to write: how I was experiencing any eddying of focus, any wandering of attention, the common language my partner and I and our various therapists and most people generally use for conceptualizing ADHD. Starting this way would be honoring my ADHD, if not necessarily celebrating it, and would feel comfortable for me. It still feels comfortable, even with a ghost interrupting and doing its (un)existential stuff.

My novel is nominally about (and narrated by) a 30-something woman called to be a ghost medium—nhập xác is the viet-language term she's given—and what that might mean in her particular bedeviled outpost of the viet refugee diaspora, Maryland, East Coast US. It's a lot of figuring without much figuring out. In one chapter, she sits up all night in a small

Are you our family? Maybe that's why I can feel you. Can you help me find him? He feels so close, especially when I talk to you. You must know him. Can you take me to him? I want to help him, and her. I think I'm clearing in Orange County waiting to commune supposed to with a ghost that never shows. That's not exactly a microcosm of the larger novel—she does end up communing with plenty of ghosts—but things never come easy, or clearly. Later on she meets an older viet auntie who laments ingesting a rare variant of aloe famed for its libido-boosting properties, foraged out in the desert somewhere by her viet shaman husband. They eat the aloe but three days later, alas, no hot sex; he's still soft as a marshmallow, and, surprise side effect, they haven't been able to fall asleep the whole time. ("Wide awake!")

Clearly it's not an exact science. None of what my narrator is trying to find and learn and preserve is. Mediumship and spirit practice and shamanism aren't exact or science. That's been my experience, too. The shaman story is a true story! He was brilliant and he was fallible, and neither quality canceled out the other. Maybe the opposite. Like the narrator of my novel, I grew up in a viet refugee family surrounded by a whole world of life (and unlife, I guess you'd call the ghosts) that was invisible to everyone else I knew, and not something we talked about away from family. A world inside the world, or beyond the world. But I only caught glimpses. It was generational, and now, as I'm reaching middle age, so much of what my mom's generation carried with them from Vietnam to the US seems to be leaving the world as they do.

Which has what, exactly, to do with ADHD?

I don't think anyone in this time knows they are meant for each

I'm not entirely sure yet. But something.

Quick story.

In my day job, I pass for a mild-mannered curator at the Smithsonian. Not too long ago, a supervisor asked me: "Lawrence, there are standards that govern everyone at this Institution; why do you think you don't have to follow them?" *Huh* was my first reaction—had I said that and forgotten? I have a big mouth and a bad memory, but not that bad, so no. Didn't I actually think that, though? I mean, it's true, I don't believe in institutions. I generally subscribe to Fred Moten's notion that the only ethical relationship to an institution is a criminal one. I remember the same supervisor once telling me, "Our first loyalty has to be to the Smithsonian," and the look on my face must've been close to the look on the face of a college student who's asked, "Does your university care about you?"

The proper response to both is "Are you fucking kidding me?" I'm familiar with the latter because I tagged along over the last seven or eight years when my wife, while writing her book *dear elia: Letters from the Asian American Abyss* (Duke University Press, 2024), posed the question above to undergrads all across the country. If you think a single student said yes, perhaps you also think people were cool with the Smithsonian making off with the remains of their elders in the early twentieth century. If the Smithsonian being founded on colonial plunder wasn't enough to wither any misplaced loyalties, there's the recent revelation that a not-inconsiderable portion of the Institution's collections of human remains, including human brains, was taken without consent for decades from mostly Indigenous and Black communities, sometimes by actual cover-of-night grave robbing; many thanks, relentless *Washington Post* reporting, for bringing these white supremacist ghoul-histories to public attention. Institutional violence is the air we breathe. That said, I realized that fateful afternoon that my dissidence was mostly postural. I couldn't credit myself with any active program to destabilize the Institution by deciding not to follow its rules. I pretty consistently did what I was told.

How . . . then . . . could I explain to this supervisor why I
supposedly thought something I didn't actually think?
My   long   pause
                    was received as defiance, which, fair enough.
Supervisor rephrased the question: "What do you call it when rules are made
for everyone and you can't follow them?"

"I call it ableism," I said before realizing I was saying it.

If you'd asked me before, I would have said yes, of course, institutions are tacitly and inherently ableist, and probably do demand neurotypicality, and do police any deviations, and have barely the faintest if any sense of ranging cognitive modes and pathways and capacities (much less a desire to better understand them, provide support across that range, begin to imagine the possibilities of an interconnected cooperative of differential)— okay, we're obviously getting into the realm of high fantasy, no sense going any further. My point is, I generally knew the above, but I hadn't guessed that my own brand of neurodivergence would ever pop up on the institutional radar and run afoul of baseline bureaucratic expectations. I'd thought I could keep amiably passing. I'm still not sure what rules I may have unwittingly broken because they routed through systems that my ADHD-blessed / ADHD-addled brain had trouble navigating.

Could I have just asked? I could have. But were the rules really at issue? Or was the crux the presumption of a neurotypical workforce for whom bureaucratic systems should never pose any trouble? The former is an easy fix; the latter is a gaping chasm. I find it unlikely that in 2023 a major institution and its various officers and managers could really fathom, let alone admit the existence of, that chasm. Bad faith is the essence of ableism.

*

For the narrator of my novel, and for me, the prospect of listening to ghosts begins with the unavoidable realities of limited capacities and limited access: no teachers (or at least willing teachers) of mediumship anywhere to be found, and my viet is terrible. My narrator and I can form a picture based on hearing a few stories, but that's barely a pencil sketch of the social and epistemological conditions in which my mom's generation was raised in VN.

I grew up on the East Coast of the US, first on the traditional lands of the

Alachua, Timucua, Seminole, and Potano peoples, now known as Gainesville, FL, and later on the traditional territory of the Piscataway Nation, now known as PG County, Maryland. Neither place had sizable viet communities to speak of at the time, but even if I'd grown up in one of the various viet ethnic enclaves in the US, I still would've had far less exposure to ghost and healing and shamanic and oracular or other fortune-telling traditions than my mom did in prewar VN. My mom once told me that the severed leg of a ghost "really" walked back and forth past the foot of her bed when she was a kid. So much exists inside that "really." She never would've had to append it back in her hometown of Tây Ninh. It's a plea, a filter, a turbulence, a closing door, a wound. Put another way: my mom and I and most of the non-viet neighbors and classmates I grew up around had radically different baseline conceptions of what is knowable and possible.

Does that possibly extend to mean we had fundamentally different neurologies?

As a preeminent non-neuroscientist, someone without a lick of expertise about the brain, it seems to me that yes, our brains were not exactly the same. Not when it came to a vast cognitive domain of engagements—social and phenomenological and physiological and on and on—with ghosts and a whole wide and wild universe of unbeing and beyond-life. I'm picturing our respective brains side by side in a dark lab, lighting up very differently under ghost stimuli, signaling our widely diverging neural capacities and networks and pathways.

Am I suggesting that ghost practice and experience constitute a form of neurodivergence?

No, that's not my claim to make. . . . It's overreaching, and maybe-possibly-probably offensive to neurodivergent folks and ghost practitioners alike.

But I do want to gently nudge the cookie to the middle of the table and leave it there.

I think

I know you !
I think you're like me!
That's why I can feel him in
you. And mama too. That's
wonderful. Let's
go find

Okay, this ghost message and the others above don't come from me, I should mention. They're not messages I imagined, or channeled, or overheard, here in this essay or in the novel. I asked others to channel the ghosts for me, viet diasporic writers and poets and artists and scholars: the very generous and venturesome Matt Huynh, Cathy Linh Che, Bao Phi, Monique Truong, erin Khuê Ninh, Khôi Nguyên Trinh, Duy Đoàn, Hoa Nguyen, Mimi Thi Nguyen, Ocean Vuong, and Quế-Lâm Huỳnh, plus my loving partner Mimi Khúc. And our three kids. I know, I owe them all a lot. The process I set for myself: I don't get to ask questions about the ghosts or edit them in any way. They just have to appear in the world of the novel, and my narrator has to coexist with them, figure out how to make sense of them, or sometimes live with the distinct possibility of not being able to. Abdicating my ability to directly write or rewrite the book's ghosts restricts my capacities to decide their choices or script their relationships to the world of the novel. My narrator can respond to them, and speculate about them, and have feelings in response to whatever they choose to say, but without real measures of control or understanding. Such a relationality, I want to think, is consonant with how I've always encountered ghosts and ghost practice in my lived (and dreaming) experience. Ghosts show up when and how they choose, most often inconveniently, and say and do what(ever the fuck) they want. Maybe interrupting the easy surface of your life is part of the point. And if you can't really tell ghosts what to do, and can't really understand them and their operation in our world of the living, then marking those limitations should be a starting point for writing about them. The limitations should be threaded into the language, and even into the process.

Ceding this kind of control feels beautiful to me.
Why do we think we're I entitled to it, in our
writing and otherwise? feel more Or that it's
always a good real right now. thing? It seems to
me a very potentially maybe I'm more colonial impulse, and
an ableist one, real when there to insist upon dominion
over 's more knowing
and direction. To grief not be willing to
humble ourselves before the unknown.
To not be able to accept and love our limitations.

I wanted the process of creating the novel to be one of naming limitations. I wanted the process of asking viet friends and family and admired colleagues and writers and thinkers to channel ghosts, and then of me building the novel around those ghosts, to be one of trying to understand what it would take, and look like, to make peace with what you didn't and couldn't know, with due reverence to the unknown and unknowable.

You could call it a *human* process, understood to be flawed and fallible. I wanted to conceive of it as a *living* one: a process with all the complexity and indeterminacy of my own lived experience, one that could grow and change, and move without me moving it, even get turned all around by the unexpected. A process that could exist at least partly outside of my control, in some complex interrelation with
a surrounding world.
But human and living weren't quite right. I was writing about ghosts, after all. My process had to make room for the dead, the after-death, the beyond-life, too. I was grasping for some of what lies beyond my understandings of life, a process of creation open to possibility beyond my small senses of possibility and openness, grounded as both are in the fine grain of the time and place in which I exist. This wouldn't be somehow abandoning

the contours (that are also the limitations) of my life and imagination, but illuminating them, putting them in new conversation, appreciating them anew. Baldwin going to Paris to learn what it means to be an American. Venturing into the afterlife to better understand life. Something along these lines has been my ludicrously romantic, or romantically ludicrous, hope for the process of creating the novel.

Approaching the novel as a communal project was also me trying to opt out of the abiding literary myth of individualism. We keep telling ourselves that reading and writing and the beautiful writing life are, at heart, solitary endeavors. Good solitary. Sublime solitary. But isolation isn't always good. We want it to be necessary time with ourselves, time away from the devouring world, and it can be. But please remember,

isolation is also a lowest common denominator tactic of repressive
regimes across regions and histories. Kundera's injunction: "The struggle
of man against power is the struggle of memory against forgetting." Our struggle as writers and readers is to hold on to the memory of violent struggle against totalitarian governments

—especially as those governments continually produce historical
amnesia,

make us forget, hide away their brutalizing operations of
gathering

and consolidating power. The memory Kundera speaks of is
not individual but *collective* memory,

operating across lifetimes and landscapes—
and for refugees, across seascapes, and for ghosts
and those who would commune
with ghosts, across the boundaries between

life and death. Forgetting
contains memory in the

small room of a single life. Or a sanitarium. Or a diagnosis, including
ADHD.

Rendering us or convincing us to render ourselves alone in all the many ways possible. Atomizing populations has always been a wedge tactic du jour, or let's say instead wedge tactic đặc biệt, for preempting or

breaking apart the kinds of collectives and coalitions and unions and revolutions that agitate for the rights that regimes would prefer never to grant. We have to be wary of any structures, myths, or sweet supportive messages pushing us to be solitary in ways that just happen to maintain existing systems of power and governance. And if the choice *is* isolation, at the very least
let's figure out how to isolate together.

To my supervisor that day I said,

> The idea that one set of rules should work for a wide range
> of people with very different bodyminds, different needs and capacities,
> and that those who have any trouble conforming to a set of rules built
> with some nonexistent person's capacities in mind should be faulted for it:
> that's ableism. It's unfair, and violently so. It not only demands an impossible
> conformity but asks everyone to invisibilize our differences—
> and exempt ourselves from being responsible for
> helping one another.

I'm pretty sure that for the supervisor, this all amounted to a big balloon of hot air and futile sounds. It was still worth enunciating. If it sounds sanctimonious, maybe it was, but my personal feeling is that sanctimony flows sideways or down, rarely uphill.

A central imperative of disability justice is making visible
differential engagements with our physical and
sensory worlds and naturalizing our varying
needs—counter to how those needs are
commonly pathologized. The point is troubling
the smoothed surface of universal experience,
the received idea that there is a normal
range of capacities and needs from which the sick
and wounded and disabled may temporarily,
and frustratingly, stray, but to which they can (be made to) return.
Particularly for the purposes of properly contributing

to society as workers and buyers and taxpayers.
Ableism requires us to uphold this
insupportable fantasy, and avoid noting the
inconsistencies that fray its edges, *fuck, shouldn't I squeeze*
in a few extra hours at the office before
my sextuple bypass heart surgery tomorrow morning?
In which case shouldn't the employees I
oversee be able to at least respond to emails faster?
A central nonsensicality of the myth of the normal healthy
human: we are all dying some every day.
But forget that. Forget the awful toll of forgetting that.
Forget better. Ableism is a lot of self-abnegating
and everyone else-abnegating, policing outwards and inwards,
gaslighting, shame, and terrible.

In place of the ableist imperative to be well,
disability justice offers interdependence and communal
care. Pause for homage to three of my dear colleagues at
the World's Largest Museum and Research
Complex over roughly the last decade,
Adriel Luis, Kālewa Correa, and Nafisa Isa,
with whom I was blessed to be interdependent. As
a group we learned together to say no thank you to
singular service to an institution and, instead, yes
to a kind of plural service through and beyond it— to the
peoples and communities and lands and waters
institutions are nominally founded to serve. And each other.
Plural as in collaborative, cooperative, grounded in
values of co-governance and co-ownership,
accountability, collective well-being.
Plural as in centering process and relationships,
broadening access, continually reconfirming
consent, continually listening and
learning . . .

Can we not embrace these forms of interdependence in the literary arts? Can we not write and build literary spaces in ways that intentionally foster healthy and equitable relationships across vast differences of all stripes and shapes? Can we not grow and draw from one another, recognize one another's limitations and capacities beyond some arbitrarily near shore of "normal" ? Create not by absenting our needs but channeling through them, with them, for them, for one another?

Ableism is baked into how we've come to understand every layer of literature, literary writing, and literary life. I can only offer a modest starting point from here in my little village of ADHD, pointing urgently, as I write, up toward the much larger, much-needed survey of neurodivergent writers and readers all over, the legion of angry villagers amassing on a hill above. Once we start asking and listening in earnest, there'll be no shortage of articulations of how our literary arts field is failing the neurodivergent. Some of those folks will first need help, as I did, to understand and trace outlines of their neurodivergence. That the field itself is not equipped to give them any of that support is one more dimension of its ableism. Gratitude to the good folks at Zoeglossia and Milkweed's Multiverse imprint and Unrestricted Interest among other organizations and projects for hauling open that door, beginning the good work of creating a disabled literary arts community and demanding disability justice in and through literature. (A large portion of the positive energy in this essay comes from a life- and neurodivergent arts–affirming Zoom call I had with Chris Martin of Multiverse and Unrestricted Interest last year, the likes of which I wish for neurodivergent writers and readers everywhere. Go read Chris's work and plug into his projects—that way lies care, resources, vision, and fun stuff.)

There are so many uncritically accepted presumptions about writing in terms of organization, register of language, affect, what the writing looks like on the page and the sentence level, the sensory experience of it, what thinking and feeling can look like or how they can manifest on the page, how they can manifest as generative friction between page and reader. How experience with the world can appear on the page, and "appear" is a bad descriptor. All shot through and through with unexamined ableism. Same goes, sadly, for what counts as a writing process and what constitutes a writing life, as well as the systems and infrastructures comprising the literary arts field.

*

A favorite poem of mine, “Corruption” by Srikanth Reddy, winds to a close with a little-known, wondrous oddity—that the cuttlefish, used for thousands of years to make sepia ink, glows for several days when it dies. “You can read by this light,” the poem ends.

About two years ago, I started using an adapted version of the line in my biographical note: “Sometimes you can see new things by the light of his ADD.” It was my first small public act of claiming neurodivergence. A nod to a poet and thinker I greatly admire, it was also intended to be a little funny, a little mournful. I wanted to ask someone meeting me and my work for the first time to view my neurodivergence as a part of who I am, how I encounter the world, and I guess, per the function of the short bio genre, why I might be considered to matter.

It comes at the end of my bio, following a few opening lines, pretty standard across the arts and academia, outlining my institutional affiliations, highest-profile accomplishments and publications to date, maybe a prestigious accolade or two. All of which signal who I am professionally. All of which, also, are calibrated to perfunctorily obliterate so much of what makes me who I am as a writer, artist, scholar, curator, editor, organizer, mentor, teacher, student, and, first and finally, reader. Maybe none of these identities really make sense to me any more without neurodivergent prefixed, and all are, naturally, inseparable from who I am as a son, partner, father, friend, dumbass, world historically great ice cream maker, colleague, companion, and forlorn and bewildered-looking fellow passenger on DC’s Green Line Metro some weekday evenings. How was my bio ever actually my bio before? This line was the first speck of my humanity I allowed into it.

What a reminder: sometimes the person who can see new things by the light of your ADHD is you. I made zero progress on my novel for ten years until I embraced a writing process that was consonant with not only what I wanted to write about but also my ways of knowing and not-knowing as a mixed viet neurodivergent child of a refugee family of healers and doctors, grapefruit lip balm–weight loss hucksters, NASA and NIH scientists, and ghost practitioners. A process fashioned with my limits of knowing as guideposts all along the way. Then I wrote the whole damn first draft in a few hallucinatory bursts, and it felt better and righter than writing ever has to me. Because for the first time it took into account, I permit myself to take into account, my own cognitive and emotional and ethical needs, in some balance, I hope, with the needs of those in community around me. Living and dead. I humbly offer up the book and its process as a strange and fierce and lovingly backward-ass alternate model for how to write through one's neurodivergence, not through sublimating it.

Also: being chewed up by institutional machinery by/for the blinking light of my ADHD has shown me what happens to the ethical wiring of perfectly mediocre people enlisted to be middle managers of institutions. That's a fate I've since decided it's best to avoid, despite the weak siren calls of higher pay, loftier status, and cessation of ableist abuse. ("Stop receiving, start doling out!") The only way to exist within such spaces, if one feels one has to stay, which this one has, for far too long, is to foster interdependence and embrace communal care.

Another alternate model of being I offer for consideration, less humbly in this case. I believe it's the best and only future for the literary arts as it exists now, in dire and woeful imbalance across an ecosystem that can squint and almost believe it's stewarding a precious art form, deepening social empathy, etc., etc.—bookstores and nonprofit spaces, literary centers and reading series and lit festivals, university presses and big and indie publishing houses, MFA programs and residency and retreat spaces, lit mags and funding bodies and on and on. A future via disability justice would give us a literary arts field: (1) working in cooperative coordination across levels and sectors; (2) committed to hearing and meeting the needs of the many, centering the disabled whose needs, historically, have least been met; (3) stewarded and governed by a representative body that truly represents the demographic breadth of its constituency, with real decision-making power vested for the first time in disabled leadership; and (4) attuned to excavating and redressing all of our awful, hidden inheritances of ableism as they are striated through our field and imported through literature and literary arts programming and productions and education throughout society. Key emphasis on that last part. The literary arts field is not simply ableist to a rotten core, including fundamentally violent to neurodivergent peoples working throughout it; it is centrally complicit in reproducing ableism and neurotypicality writ large, functioning as a feeder system that perennially shapes how we tell ourselves stories about who we were and are and can be, and teach future generations to tell and listen to stories about who we were and are and can be.

Most especially, as literary writers and arts administrators and stewards otherwise concerned with the soul and responsibilities of the literary arts, it is incumbent upon us to remember: we are never just ourselves, responsible for only ourselves, beholden to only ourselves. Isolation is a myth. Refusing interdependence never removes the consequences of your choices on untold others around you and to come; it simply ignores responsibility
for them. I've learned this through the light of my ADHD. Or I should say, I've learned this from the ghosts I could see by the light of my ADHD, or hear, or better to say, sense, or better still to say, perceive by extrasensory capacity, by the figurative
light-glow-illumination-signal, or the call to
pay attention, of my ADHD.

Ghosts visit us if we make ourselves safe to be visited. Or sometimes they just do what they want. I can't claim to know for sure—and I feel comfort,
and
find calm and release, in that not-knowing. That knowing should rest with

ghosts, and if my uncles and aunts and mom and the generations before
them
got to share in some luminous portion of it, maybe someday a portion will
come to me, or someone else, some future generation. Or not, depending,
I can hope, on the balance of needs of an ecosystem beyond the few, beyond
the rich and powerful, beyond those who believe there is such a thing as a
normal, healthy person. Beyond those who willfully forget about most of the
rest of us, about the hurting and dying nature of all of us, about our dead and
their world and its needs, about all of what exists outside the small domain
of what we think we know and get to control. Maybe via my novel,
ghosts can remind some readers of these things. For literature and the
literary
arts more broadly, there can be no maybes. The two must always bear the
responsibility of opening the vast possibilities of thinking and feeling
our everyday world continually forecloses. Maybe ghosts can visit us if
our literatures help us become safer to visit. Without question, the prospect
of visiting ourselves, the deep interior spaces we let languish, is most
viable when the literary arts field reminds us why we need to, and
when our literatures help us reimagine
ourselves as safer visitors: more tender and caring, better able to
encounter difference and not-knowing, gentler with our own and one
another's limitations. These are all euphemisms for disability justice
principles, and with shared commitment, we can infuse these generosities
and humilities into our reading and writing, our reading practices, and
writing processes, our literary arts spaces and infrastructures,
our publishing and education systems and beyond.
I'll stop jabbering and let someone else, something else,
have the closing floor of this page
because in
that sense, too, we can be plural, refuse
isolation, write by not-writing , by
listening-collaborating ,
hold space for ways of knowing
and being other than ou—

I think I've
been here
with you
, in and out, this
whole journey. I hope so
. I like that idea. I wonder
if grief shapes
your being
too . maybe it's some
thing else since you're
there and I'm here
and we in terlace in
ebbs and flows,
eddies ofconnection
in our wake

PROMPT: By the Light of *Your* ADHD

Sometimes the person who can see new things by the light of your ADHD is you. What would it mean to approach your writing with this permission: to really and truly, genuinely and carefully take into account your own needs, cognitive and emotional and ethical? To embrace a writing process that is consonant with not only what you want to write about, but also the ways you encounter the world as a neurodivergent writer, reader, and human?

1. Start with your needs. What do you need in order to be ready to write? These needs could be big, small, physical, emotional, temporal, or related to a kind of desk/chair, a noise level, or childcare—any and everything. Make a list.
2. Consider your writing process and the degree to which it currently meets those needs. If they aren't always being met, why not? If they are, is that arrangement sustainable, including in the event of major life changes? Do you have friends, family, or colleagues you could call upon for help? Or depending on your capacity, could you offer something like reciprocal support to writers with whom you are in community?
3. Now let's think specifically about your ADHD. Does your experience of it make any appearances in the list you made in step 1? On top of making your writing possible, naming and naturalizing ADHD-related needs can be truly freeing and validating. Building upon that, let's consider how your ADHD might serve as a resource for your writing, a guide—a light. Consider the ways it shapes your bodymind's encounters with the world around you. Can you identify several specific features or elements of your ADHD? What can any of these illuminate in terms of how you write, or maybe even why?

4. For an upcoming writing project, try this little experiment: Pick a feature or element of your ADHD you identified in step 3. Now "point" it at the project—whatever feels right, whether a word or sentence, emotional current or character, bit of plotting or scene-setting. Or to pan further back, think about your goals for the project, the audiences you might have in mind, or the process you've laid out to write it. What would it mean to reapproach any one of those things with this feature or element of your ADHD in mind? How might doing so open up new possible choices or directions? How might it shift how you *feel* about the act of writing? Now repeat with other elements, and don't look back.

11

Non-Standard Operating Procedure

ELIZABETH ITO

A few minutes ago, I was washing the dishes when I shouted, "DRUG DOGS! ANECDOTE ABOUT DRUG DOGS!" And then I laughed because I am the only person in the house. My husband is at work and my kids are at school.

I yelled this because I suddenly remembered a bombshell revelation I had a couple of hours ago. At the time, I told myself to stop putting away the laundry and go write it down, but I didn't, and then I promptly forgot about it. As I worked through the dishes, I had the sense that there had been a momentary crucial thought I'd wanted to put into this essay—but I couldn't recall what it was. And then it came to me: the drug dogs. This time I *did* manage to write it down.

Several years ago, while on a flight, I overheard a man telling his seatmate about his line of work. He said that he trained police dogs to sniff out drugs and other contraband. He then explained that the kinds of dogs that work best for that purpose have to be "a little bit crazy." They need to be completely obsessed with their task in a way that other dogs aren't. It made so much sense to me. I have ADHD, and my own neuro-atypical traits—from obsessive hyperfocus on projects to unusual approaches to storytelling and problem-solving—have been the keys to my success. They have helped me to build a career as an animator, writer, director, and creator of an award-winning animated series.

City of Ghosts

In 2019 Netflix hired me and a handful of other young creatives to help build a new studio, Netflix Animation. They tasked us with creating our own animated projects and developing a studio that would be an appealing place for animation artists to work. They wanted the studio and the content produced there to be wildly innovative and to attract every possible kind of artist and subscriber. They also invited us to think outside the box when it came to the projects we brought to the table. What kind of show would you make if you could make whatever you wanted, and have it be any length you wanted, with the thought that people might also watch it in any order they wanted? Typically, television is beholden to predetermined airtime lengths (a half-hour to hour-long format), and on network television, there are built-in breaks for commercials. On a streaming service like Netflix, you don't have any of those limitations. Additionally, Netflix was playing with how to bring different kinds of interactive storytelling to the platform, such as Choose Your Own Adventure narratives. This opened up a whole new way to think about telling a story—could the viewer feel more involved in the story, somehow, beyond just watching? There were a lot of opportunities to do things differently, and it was up to us to figure out what we could do with those opportunities.

I ended up creating *City of Ghosts*, a six-episode animated series set in Los Angeles and using an unusual set of components—scripted and unscripted, historical and fictional, photographic and drawn. The show follows a little girl named Zelda, who has a "ghost club" in which she and her friends find out about local history by talking to ghosts and the people who live in their neighborhoods. Unlike most traditional animated series for kids, *City of Ghosts* is presented in a documentary format, combining interviews with real people with the fictional ghost club, kid-character narrative. The dialogue for both children and adults was kept at a slow, natural pace, leaving room for pauses and moments for thinking, a pace that reflects reality more than most American cartoons.

Before *City of Ghosts*, I had started blending photographs and animation in a short I made called *Welcome to My Life*. It was about my brother and my family, but I turned them into monster characters trying to live a regular life in a normal human world. I used photographic backgrounds with animated characters because I wanted to make people feel as if these characters existed in real life. *City of Ghosts* was a continuation of that visual idea and style. For the backgrounds of our show, we combined photographs with both 2D and 3D animation, composited in a way that blended the three techniques together to create a look that continues to surprise people when they discover it, mostly because they can't figure out why the image they're looking at is so real, but also very different from reality.

City of Ghosts is groundbreaking in its look, sound, and style of storytelling, but it also confronts topics that aren't typically covered in mainstream programming for children. During the interviews with real people that helped us tell the historical pieces of the show's stories, I tried to leave room for people to tell the whole truth of their lives, even when the conversation veered into topics that are hard to talk about with children, like when Atomic Nancy reflects on Japanese internment and how the incarceration of her family during that time affected her as a child. It was something that came up naturally in the interview, and it reflected important context for her character. Other episodes bring up the genocide of the Tongva people, gentrification and cultural diversity in LA neighborhoods, immigrant communities and Indigenous languages, and LGBTQIA representation.

The show also succeeded in being told from the perspective of a marginalized point of view, rather than a dominant, mainstream media point of view. All of these topics are presented in a way that's relatable for children. Children are the main characters in the show, the ones asking the questions, and adults are confronted with having to answer truthfully. Anyone who has kids or works with kids on a regular basis knows how good children are at asking questions that make adults uncomfortable. I wanted to reflect that unpredictability in my show, but also use it as an opportunity to open up the narrative and include the historical struggles and injustices that my ancestors, and the ancestors of many other people in the United States, have experienced.

Since the project was a hybrid of fiction and documentary, there were a number of ways that our production process was different. Instead of collaborating with a team of children's television writers, I collaborated with documentary writers and researchers. I wanted to use actual photographs of locations rather than having a designer paint them, so we looked for a photographer who had the kind of background and skills that would be right for a show about Los Angeles, and we found Kwasi Boyd-Bouldin, an immensely talented street photographer and artist, who grew up all over Los Angeles around the same time as I did. Typically, in an animated show, you are legally required to hire voice actors who are represented by the Screen Actors Guild. I found a way to circumvent this requirement for my show, because I wanted the characters to sound like real people, not professional actors, and to do that I had to hire non-actors.

City of Ghosts was the only show to come out of Netflix Animation that won a Peabody Award. It succeeded because I did exactly what the studio asked me to do: I created a show in a new way about something that was different from what anyone, anywhere, was making. To create a show that delivered all that took a lot of work. Whenever I wanted to do something in a way that wasn't the standard procedure, it took a lot of explaining to the people in charge of budgets and hiring, many meetings, and a fair amount of anxiously waiting to see if I could get permission to do things my own weird way. When I wanted to hire a documentary writer instead of a children's television writer, I had to have a number of meetings in order to get approval, since no one on the animation side of the company had ever set up a production to include a role like that. Similarly, when we were recording interviews with real people for the show, there were at least three different times when a new lawyer was brought into the studio, and I had to explain why our show wasn't using union actors. In all of these nonstandard approaches, I did things in a way that made sense to me, but that went against much of the accepted wisdom about how to work in television.

The Front of the Room

As a child, I loved drawing and making up stories. The first really memorable ones were mostly about mice who wore clothes and slept in matchbox beds inside the walls. Sometimes the stories were about turtles or our cat. As I got older, I used my creativity to express myself and to help me work through whatever I was thinking about or feeling. If I was mad at someone, I'd draw a picture about it.

I still make art and tell stories for similar reasons, and I love what I do. The process of making stories for entertainment, however, involves not only drawing and writing, and coming up with ideas, but also presenting the concept to the studio in a pitch. As a storyboard artist, I had to learn how to get up in front of a room full of people, point to my drawings and writing on a board, and, if necessary, act out what was happening in the story. In a pitch, sometimes you're telling jokes that you're hoping people (often a bunch of your friends) will think are funny. When you're done, everyone critiques it and gives you feedback, usually requiring a lot of additional follow-up work to address everyone's thoughts. Sometimes you will present the same sequence so many times that you end up remembering the dialogue and jokes for the rest of your life. As a person who would get nervous simply raising my hand to speak in class as a kid, I'm not really sure how I got myself into a line of work that requires so much public speaking.

When I had to present my project to Netflix Animation Studios at an all-staff meeting, I was so nervous that I ran to the bathroom before I was supposed to go on and spent fifteen minutes holding the armpits of my shirt under the hand dryer. I had sweated through them while waiting to go onstage. Much to my surprise, when I ran into a colleague the day after, he said I did a great job during my presentation and that I seemed totally relaxed. Observations like this one catch me off guard because that's not at all how I feel on the inside. My colleague had no idea how much work I had done to get to a point where I didn't outwardly seem nervous.

When I used to play piano in high school, there were a couple of times during practice recitals where I hit a minor mistake, then completely forgot how to get back into a piece I'd memorized. Sometimes I was so stuck that another student had to bring my sheet music up for me to find my place. This was mortifying, but I kept learning piano because I liked it and I was good at it. I had to teach myself tricks so that my nervousness and fear of performing for an audience wouldn't completely immobilize me. I made sure to practice starting pieces I was playing from multiple spots, so that if I made a mistake while playing from memory, I would have other places that I knew I could start from, should I experience a memory block. My teacher would have a number of low-pressure "practice performances" scheduled for me, in front of family and friends. The benefit was that I could get used to the feeling of performing and learn how to manage my anxiety with tricks like bringing hand warmers if my hands got cold, or practices like breathing and grounding to help calm my nerves and mentally get in the zone while I was waiting for my turn to perform. It also helped me to record myself playing, not for sharing with others but to know how I sounded and looked onstage. This helped me learn how to be more intentional with my performance and body language. Many of these tricks are the same ones I've come to rely on while pitching storyboards and shows. Most of my tricks really have to do with learning to be in front of people, knowing that there might be unexpected hiccups, but that I can train myself to not let them stop me in my tracks. Looking back, I now see that this could also be a form of teaching myself to mask—to hide ADHD differences from the world.

Sublimation for the Win

After I completed *City of Ghosts* and had time to reflect on the experience of running my own weird show, I realized that a lot of the things I've achieved in my career, while fulfilling, have also come at a price. They have increased my stress and anxiety levels and, consequently, my cholesterol and blood pressure. I often find myself asking, "Why am I even doing this if it's stressing me out so much?" I knew there were some things I needed to better understand about the way my brain works if I wanted to continue to take on higher-level jobs without wrecking my health and my self-esteem. That's when I came across ADHD.

When I first started to read about ADHD, I immediately connected to everything being described. I devoured books and internet articles, because I found a lot of advice on the topic to be helpful for me. In an article about people with a high IQ and ADHD, I read, "Those who grow up celebrated as 'smart' internalize their intellect as a foundation of their identities and a source of self-esteem. They know that they carry the expectation of success. Thriving in school with little effort, they have been told that success will be theirs."[1]

For most of my life so far, as a child who was identified as gifted and talented in grade school, I thought the things I struggled with were because I was secretly lacking in some way, and my internal voices would convince me of it: "You're just not that smart. You aren't that good at playing piano—you should just quit. You'll probably embarrass yourself in front of everyone." I think it would've made it easier to understand a lot of the challenges I felt inside, that weren't reflected outwardly, if I'd known more about what ADHD was.

One more piece of the puzzle came into focus for me when I came across the term "sublimation" in a list of ADHD attributes from the

1 Ellen Littman, "'I'm Smart, So I Should Be Able to Overpower ADHD. Right?'" *ADDitude*, updated July 11, 2022, https://www.additudemag.com/high-iq-and-adhd-high-functioning/.

American Psychological Association: "A defense mechanism in which unacceptable sexual or aggressive drives are unconsciously channeled into socially acceptable modes of expression and redirected into new, learned behaviors, which indirectly provide some satisfaction for the original drives."[2]

I think sublimation is perhaps responsible for the direction my work has taken in the animation industry and belies what I hope to achieve with it. As I learn more about inequity, marginalized and misunderstood communities, climate change, and the myriad things we're confronted with as civilization evolves over time, I've had a lot of moments in which I question how I can help make the world better. I am only one person who makes cartoons for children for a living. To feel powerless is frustrating, and I feel angry and aggressive when I dwell on it.

But I try to channel that frustration into creative work that reflects how I feel about big issues in the world, and that does so through a personal lens. I like to talk to people and to hear the stories of where they come from. It makes me happy to learn about new places by listening to people who live there, and to preserve their voices and something about the way they see the world. I make things hoping that children will appreciate seeing themselves reflected truthfully, because I think kids should know how funny and smart they are. Selfishly, I also do what I do because I love my own kids and family so deeply. I hope I can make this world better for them and for all their friends. If I can show them the good that exists in them and also make them laugh? This drug-sniffing dog can retire as a very happy dog, indeed.

The Next New Thing

I come from a family who are curious and tend to be early adopters of new gadgets, when the gadgets are affordable on a middle-class income. We love to find new pathways and tools that allow our

2 "Sublimation," *APA Dictionary of Psychology*, updated April 19, 2018, https://dictionary.apa.org/sublimation.

creativity to blossom. We've always been interested in what people now call "life hacks": finding a new, efficient way to do a task, or repurposing something for a new use, or improving an old process with a new adaptation or tool.

Lately I'm trying out a device called the Freewrite Traveler. On this device, all I'm allowed to do is write: it has no other functions. I remember seeing a hipster at a café using one of these, an earlier, chunkier model. I definitely cracked some jokes about it. And now here I am, no better than a Starbucks hipster man from 2013. It's essentially a digital typewriter, but less bulky and eye-catching. It's better designed for, well . . . traveling. The screen only shows a portion of what you've typed and is minimally editable. People in the reviews complain about how laggy it is, but I'm not too sensitive about that. The display is very basic, and the interface is such that I can't quickly click away to peek at social media, look up something on the internet, or check email.

I bought this gadget because I was looking for something to lessen the chances that I would get distracted by that ever-present temptation, the infinite universe of the internet. But also, since I'm old (okay, middle-aged), a little bit lazy about reading instructions and remembering key commands, and very new to using this thing, it's also pretty much impossible for me to go back and make edits. That's been great, because it forces me to keep moving forward rather than getting stuck perfecting and making micro adjustments before I'm done. When I use it out and about, I hope someone is making fun of me, laughing at this hipster trying way too hard, using an old-fashioned tool to improve their productivity in this distraction-in-your-pocket world.

Oh, You Wanted This . . . Typed?

Right now, I find myself on an airplane trying to finish writing this essay on my Freewrite Traveler. Of course I've waited until the very last minute, why wouldn't I? Procrastination is one of the traits of ADHD that when I first came across it, I felt it in my bones. Waiting until the final minute to do things is part of the adventurousness and thrill-seeking trait of ADHDers. It probably also explains why, despite being mostly an introvert, there is a part of me that loves the risk of creating for an audience.

When I'm writing or creating, I have a million ideas all at once flying around in the air, and I hope I can catch one and use it. But where do you even put ideas after you've caught them, so that you don't then forget about them later? And how do you communicate all the idea threads in a concise way that the people who need to understand them will understand? I've collected many blank journals and books over time, with every intention of each one becoming the answer to my new organized life (that inevitably starts tomorrow). Some I bought because I liked the paper, others because of some template I was sold on momentarily.

While I was making *City of Ghosts*, I tried out many different note-taking apps—a process of trial and error that often led to unproductive, forgotten, or airdropped-into-the-void PDFs. When I first started submitting rough outlines for my show, I tried sending executives a handwritten outline for the pilot episode of *City of Ghosts*. I wrote it in a note-taking app that I was enjoying using on my iPad. My outline described where I thought the episode would go, but it was entirely scribbled in my handwriting, with a few thumbnail sketches drawn here and there. The executives politely requested that I type it out and resend. To be clear, my handwriting isn't illegible, but upon reflection, I think that to submit the notes in this form was probably akin to me pitching the show in the form of a spoken-word poem.

Hmm. Maybe I'll try that next time.

PROMPT: A Picture About a Feeling

Drawing and writing can be a great way to access our underlying concerns, feelings, worries, and obsessions. Think about something that has happened to you that brought up strong feelings—either a recent event or an important memory from childhood. Is there a color, sound, shape, or taste you associate with it? Is there an animal, supernatural creature, imaginary place, or object that comes up in association with that memory? Write or draw something using those associations. Keep the emotions in mind but don't name them.

12

A Glitch Is Not a Glitch

RAINIE OET

1. Glitches

ADHD is and isn't a glitch. A glitch is an unanticipated feature in a human-created program, an emergent property, a dynamic happening. Our capitalist culture and politicized reality are human-created programs. Since the ADHD neurotype has always existed, it *is not* a glitch. But because ADHD can only exist as a disability inside a human-created context, it *is* a glitch.

This is a political essay, in the sense that it is about what is and what could be. This essay is about interdependence. It is about writing. It is about joy.

2. *Glitch Girl!*

At the time of writing this essay, I've just turned in edits on my first novel, *Glitch Girl!*, a middle grade novel-in-verse about a nonbinary trans girl, *J*—, at the intersection of ADHD, trauma, and her obsession with a computer game that has her building a roller coaster park.

I'd been working on the book for six and a half years, on and off. Over the process of writing *Glitch Girl!*, I felt weighed down by the immensity of the project. I couldn't imagine writing it in a way that did justice to the complexity of the true experience many neurodivergent and trans children have. So, for most of the early versions, I tried to settle for less.

Glitch Girl! is a novel composed of hundreds of short poems. When I wrote the first batch of these poems, I wrote them out of order, not knowing where they would fit, only that I was building toward *something*. As I revised the poems and wrote new ones, I moved all of the pieces around. It was through this process of restructuring that a narrative began to emerge. I then added new poems, which I again moved around. I repeated this process of adding and restructuring over and over again.

I kept thinking the book was done only to realize, months later, that it wanted to be more. First, I wrote it as a short poetry book for adults that was solely about *J—*'s (my own) obsession with a computer game. Then, I gave it linearity and added in the heartbreak of *J—*'s delusional, one-sided crush on a classmate. Then, I added *J—*'s trans experience. Then, I added relationships with family. Then, I added school and interiority for the secondary characters. Next, I gave it a plot and added in ADHD and trauma. Finally, I gave it a happy ending.

This approach to writing often mirrors my neurodivergent experience. For me, "what *is* true," "what *may* be true," and "what may *become* true" are all provisional, ever-shifting stories. My experience of ADHD is chaotic, sensitive, and expansive, so, like *J—* in *Glitch Girl!*, I often figure things out through trial and error, or by taking on new perspectives to see whether they feel true. Over the process of writing about transness in *Glitch Girl!*, I figured out that *I* was a trans woman!

I often love writing in first person because it's so immersive. By putting the reader into an idiosyncratic narrator's voice, I create an environment in which the reader is compelled to learn how to think like the narrator (i.e., to empathize with them). The experience of ADHD is itself idiosyncratic (i.e., non-normative); *Glitch Girl!* is full of exclamation points, digressions, and inconsistencies in *J—*'s experience of time and of herself. The novel *had* to be in first person—no other mode would allow readers to fully inhabit the ins and outs of *J—*'s inner life.

While *Glitch Girl!* is about a lot of things—like any childhood is—at the heart of the book is *J—*'s neurodivergence. Like the glitches that

J— loves discovering in her computer game, she believes that her ADHD is part of what makes her "silly and different and good."[1] *J—*'s ADHD is present in her revelrous joy throughout the book, her excitement, and her obsessiveness. ADHD is also a constant source of tension between *J—* and her teachers, peers, and parents. She hums during a test, taps a pencil on her desk after repeatedly being told to stop, and constantly forgets her homework. She says, "I don't know why I do things. I just realize I'm doing them, like waking up slowly at the end of a dream." She yearns to be understood but lacks the tools to understand herself: "My brain's a broken mirror, reflecting everything at once so I lose track because there's too much, and it's super hard to control myself." Sometimes, she hates herself: "The reason I'm bad is because I . . . am a glitch. I shouldn't exist."

ADHD is hard for me to write about. For one thing, for much of my life, I only knew ADHD through its negative consequences. From the time I was six, I knew I had ADHD; my mom woke me up every morning by pushing a max-dose extended-release Ritalin into my mouth so that I might not be as ADHD that day. I was punished, frequently, traumatically, at home and in school, for my "bad" behavior—and grew up believing *I* was bad. For example: my father hit me with a belt repeatedly, sometimes with the metal buckle, because I couldn't explain why I misbehaved even while on the medication. My school locked me in a tiny soundproof closet for hours because I spoke back to a teacher who was angry at me for not being able to stop jiggling my leg. So, like *J—*, I started saying to myself: "ADHD stupid brain. Maggot brain."

It is difficult for me to separate much of my experience of ADHD from my two-decade experience of being cluelessly in the closet as a traumatized trans girl. How much of my childhood acting out came from ADHD versus abuse versus living within an unwanted gender?

1 This and all other quotes from *Glitch Girl!*, copyright © 2025 by Rainie Oet, are used by permission of Kokila, an imprint of Penguin Young Readers Group, a division of Penguin Random House LLC. All rights reserved.

I just don't know. It is additionally difficult for me to separate my life-long awareness of ADHD from my recent understanding that I am also autistic.

And last, I am trying to separate my experience of neurodivergence from my experience of masking. As a weird, hyper kid who struggled with impulse control and relationships, I grew many "masks"—of emotional repression, dysphoric gender performance, perfectionistic achievement, and obsessive-compulsive rule setting—that I'm now learning how to take off.

When I talk about ADHD in this essay, I am talking about an experience that is connected to all my other experiences.

3. What ADHD Is and Is Not

I unlearn that ADHD is being "too much." I unlearn the urge to repress myself in order to be "okay" for others. I unlearn years of ingrained self-restraint, like when my parents signed me up for neurofeedback that would teach me to sit as still as possible and push down any urges for movement. I unlearn the lie that I'm intrinsically "annoying." Now, I want to sing, I want to scream, I want to be messy. I feel the force of how much I am. I know that I can never be too much. If *this* is too much, then I want to change people's minds so that no one is too much.

ADHD is . . . an eye that keeps the imprint of lightning for hours; a messy witch with a bathtub full of eels; a ghost haunted by the living; a flourishy turn at the end of a dance; a spoon-under-sink-spray of need.

I do not see ADHD as a "problem," although I was taught to think of it that way for decades. I unlearn that lesson. Like many "disabilities," ADHD is not inherently disabling. In fact, it is our rigid and unaccommodating world that creates and necessitates the idea of disability.

ADHD is . . . the jump of static to a hand from a doorknob; a brooch you wear when feeling powerful; a channel that guides water; a bite of lemon under the rain; the aching delight of a nerve in a bruise you don't remember getting; an effigy that will not burn.

I unlearn minimizing my ADHD: "Oh, that's just ADHD, an excuse for why I do what I do." But ADHD *is* my brain, is its own neurotype. Like a different style of swimming. Backstroke, not freestyle.

ADHD is . . . a year, full of new return; a radio overlapping stations; an oarfish in front of a shipwreck's mirror; a hand that touches and feels itself; many drums beating in different time; turning back at the maze end.

I unlearn wishing for my mind to become "normal" one day. I'll always have a mind that works like this, and that's a good thing.

ADHD is . . . a dream in which everything comes easily except for waking up; a machine that unspools VHS tapes into piles of connected ribbon; an ear that only works sometimes; an unlabeled rock collection; a false knot; a smudged glass museum pane for taxidermy.

I unlearn hating myself because of the abuse I got from my parents and from my school. I unlearn seeing myself as a behavioral problem rather than as a child with feelings and energy and hurt and hurt and hurt. I unlearn that I cannot be myself without causing problems.

ADHD is . . . pretending to be a siren when I yawn; a needle that kisses water; an earthworm that kisses water; a mother that kisses water; the fact of true randomness and the impossibility of programming it; a catalog of glow-in-the-dark fish of the bathypelagic sea.

I learn that I deserve to be fully understood, fully authentic, fully allowed. I learn that it can be good to be impulsive, to think out loud, to have a new overwhelming hobby every few months.

ADHD is . . . a 10,000-year-old architecture, full of locked doors and surrounded by water; an earthquake in a lighting store; an engine that runs on other engines' entropy; an epoxy dissolver; you, smiling in a mirror at night; an umbrella creating a crown of rain around a child.

ADHD distracted me, so many times, over the months of writing this essay: new friends (A, H, H, J, K, M, R) and new interests (pin collecting, bug farming, pentatonic flute). But still, I always keep writing, no matter what. I learn that I can trust my mind, trust my process. I finish the things I need to and let go of the things I don't. Finances allowing, I learn to have a relationship with creativity and productivity that is based on inner drive rather than wanting to gain economic or social capital.

ADHD is . . . the shape-shifting movement of an amoeba, agony twirling like a sprinkler hose in every second, creating rainbows; yarn rolled up and also there's a cat; a secret, true name shared by others; euphoria twirling like a sprinkler hose in every second, creating rainbows; a misplaced ant, looking for its colony.

I learn, period. Because ADHD means learning from everything that distracts me. I accept that anything may capture me completely at any time, and so I take everything seriously. Everything is worth paying attention to, just like everything is worth writing about.

ADHD is . . . trust for oneself; a teapot that whistles steam; a fwapping tail; a god of luck; a hydra kite that knows the wind best; an empathy for anything.

When I was in second grade, I won the Thanksgiving wishbone—broke off the larger piece—and the wish I made, my deal with the universe, was *Please take away my behavioral problems, take away my ADHD, and I'll give up being good at math.* I did let go of math, but I didn't lose my ADHD. It wasn't until I was almost thirty that I got to the place where I no longer wanted to lose my ADHD.

ADHD is a yes, and a yes, and a yes; a sum greater than the whole; a magnet that temporarily turns paper clips to magnets just by touching them; a lucid dream's ebullient takeoff to flight; a frog that makes a universe but is a tadpole first; a gem that emerges, geometry out of millions of years in one of the Earth's many hearts.

4. Practical Matters

In my world, and likely in yours as well, survival is contingent upon money, time, and attention. My stimulant medication helps a lot with the difficulty of living with ADHD in a world that makes ADHD a disability. Unmedicated ADHD is associated with a greater rate of suicide and addiction.[2] From both a personal and a public health perspective, I am a strong advocate for deregulating ADHD medication so it's

2 Zheng Chang et al., "Medication for Attention-Deficit/Hyperactivity Disorder and Risk for Suicide Attempts," *Biological Psychiatry* 88, no. 6 (September 15, 2020): 452–58, https://doi.org/10.1016/j.biopsych.2019.12.003; Bahadar S. Srichawla et al., "Attention Deficit Hyperactivity Disorder and Substance Use Disorder: A Narrative Review," *Cureus* 14, no. 4 (April 12, 2022), https://doi.org/10.7759/cureus.24068.

accessible to those who aren't able to continually jump through the many legal hoops required to obtain it.

But beyond medication, I also ground myself in habits and routines—containers for different kinds of energy—such as regular morning phone calls with friends, exercise hours, wake and sleep times, rest days, and more. (And then I must be careful to hold on to flexibility, lest the maintenance of these containers becomes an obsession that prevents me from really living.) For example, while actively working on *Glitch Girl!*, I tried to show up at the same time every day for however long I could. Fifteen minutes. Thirty minutes. An hour. Two hours. I made a ritual of it. After breakfast, I'd put on music and write and revise until I got tired, or bored, or had to clock into my job. What seemed like an impossibility—completing the novel—became possible only through faith and bite-size chunks of attention spread out over several years.

Living my life in the happiest way involves embracing, rather than suppressing, my constant, constantly shifting hyperfixations. *Glitch Girl!*, too, encompasses many of my childhood hyperfixations—roller coasters, video games, magnets, black holes, crystals, mood rings. As an adult, I still love going down rabbit holes. Rather than rejecting the discursiveness and obsessiveness of my fascination, I let each new interest teach me more about what it means to be human.

5. On Unmasked Interdependence

*Inter*dependence is the radical act of becoming whole by sharing responsibility for each other's well-being. This may cover co-caring for each other's emotional regulation, art-making practices, physical needs, moral direction, and autonomy.

*In*dependence, on the other hand, is capitalism's false narrative of success, i.e., "pulling yourself up by your bootstraps" or being "self-made"—it's about telling yourself you don't *need* others to survive or succeed, that you can do it all by yourself. This is a lie, of course: a lie that often lays the groundwork for the exploitation of others' physical, mental, or emotional labor. (There is no billionaire CEO without employees; there is no food without those who produce it; there are no authors without there being readers.) Autonomy (i.e., the ability to differentiate ourselves from those we are in relationship with) looks different in *inter*dependence; it simply means that we bear witness to the ways we are different, and we allow others to extend their lives beyond our own. Like watching a cloud change. Without this kind of autonomy, our lives would be stifling and exhausting: a closed system of mutual codependency. But the point of *inter*dependent autonomy is to make happiness easier for all those involved.

I've come to believe that ADHD is both deeply relational and deeply autonomous. My mind's experience of ADHD—jumping from one thing to another, getting lost in the sauce—often separates me from the flow of neurotypical conversations or situations, lending itself toward a strong feeling of individuality. And yet, existing with ADHD as a detached individual is literally impossible. My mind is always forming relationships. Connections with people and their ideas. Also, ADHD has set me up to need people. I need support with emotional regulation and executive functioning. I used to be ashamed of how much help I needed, but learning to unmask, especially with others, changed that.

Unmasking—letting myself *be* ADHD: hyper, associative, silly, and unfiltered—goes hand in hand with interdependence. We can only truly give and receive what we need from a place of mutual authenticity. In fact, I didn't realize how much I loved myself and my ADHD until I made community with other neurodivergent people, and we *unmasked together*—wiggling and singing and screaming, laughing until our sides hurt and then laughing more. Now, my need for people is a source of happiness. I've had amazing experiences giving and receiving care in the form of comforting touch, body doubling, and food preparation. This mutual unmasking has taught me how much this world, my American culture, is wrong to force the isolation of capitalistic independence. ADHD has taught me, as my transness has taught me, to speculate. To imagine that other ways of living can be better than the status quo.

I didn't seek out this community of caring weirdos. Instead, as marginalized people often do, we naturally gravitated toward each other. Many times throughout my life, I've encountered other trans people, other queer people, and other AuDHD people; however, it was only after I started to begin to accept myself, and *unmask*, that I was able to actually be receptive to *making community with* people like me. Now, almost all of my friends are neurodivergent and trans. By coincidence (or not), most of these people are also artists.

In the last section of *Glitch Girl!*, *J—* begins to develop a friendship with another trans, neurodivergent kid. *J—* learns, much later in her life than I would consider ideal, that she is not alone, and doesn't ever have to be alone, in a world that misunderstands, disables, and abuses her. I, too, learned this later than I would have wanted, and only by forming relationships with other people like me. But I did learn it, and it's maybe the most important thing I have ever learned.

This is an essay about moving from I to we. It is an essay about moving from pain to joy. From loneliness to possibility. It is an ode to the possibilities of interdependence. It is a call to action. It is a gentle hug and shoulder squeeze to those who are struggling with their ADHD right now. It is a reminder: We are all out here; we can all love and support each other; our minds may be different but they are also so similar. We have so much to teach each other. We have so much to learn from each other. We have so much joy to share: everything is spilling out of all of us, and we can't even hold it for one second. Together, we can shape worlds that do not currently exist except in our imaginations and in each other.

This is what good writing does.

We, interdependently, are good writing.

ADHD can be difficult, frustrating, and draining. And yet, midway through *Glitch Girl!*, *J—* watches a video of herself as a toddler singing: "Rock and roll is good and bad! Come rock and roll!" and then reflects: "Everyone's always told me I'm bad for not being able to control my ADHD. But in that song, I'm saying that some things that are bad are also good. Just imagine how much nicer it would be if everyone remembered that! If *I* remembered that!"

My ADHD often feels like a force of nature—powerful beyond my control and mysteriously life-giving. Through my ADHD, I feel myself to be intimately entwined with the joy and life in everything.

A crow flies through the air above me on my balcony, and the winter sun setting early is still high enough to make its wings translucent—yellow-gray instead of black. It's there and then it's gone, and part of a larger crowd that I can hear cawing and cawing above and between the rooftops of my Los Angeles neighborhood.

PROMPT: Odes to Possibility

As someone with ADHD, I often want to go big, but I am afraid to. This prompt is maximalist. I hope you'll give it a chance.

Write a series of poems that are linked in some way—by theme, form, vocabulary, or something else. Each poem can be whatever it wants to be, using various styles, lengths, or perspectives, but choose at least one thing to keep in each poem that will connect them.

> One way to link this series is by word choice. For example, generate a word bank by thinking of a random word, then another that starts with the last letter of the previous word: *Year, Radio, Oarfish, Hand, Drum, Maze End*. Make the list as long as you want. Choose two (or more) words from the list to include in each poem.

You could write just four or five poems, but I'd advise you to see how many you can write, either all at once or as an ongoing daily practice. Can you write twelve, or twenty?

> Let each poem be idiosyncratic. Maybe there is some sort of narrative, and maybe it isn't linear. Consider letting the passage of time be inconsistent within and between the poems. You might take the speaker (or speakers) from point A to points B, G, X, or Z.

Pay attention to how change is showing up in these poems as a group. Try out different relationships (mirrored, at odds, or both at different times) between internal and external change. Try putting the poems in different orders and see what happens.

> Want to go even bigger? Set your poems aside for a while; then come back and try to use them to make something else. Maybe there's a short story in there that uses some of the language from the poems. Maybe a song cycle, with the poems as libretto. Maybe they want to become a graphic novel! What else can you do with these things you've made?

13

Outside Voices

JENNIFER L. KNOX

"Next to animation, poetry is the fastest medium," one of my art school professors said. Apropos of what, and the name of the professor and the class, I don't recall.

That was either the semester I changed my major from theater to English or the semester I changed my major from English to art. Whoever the prof was, it's a testament to her teaching that I was listening at all. Most teachers, I'd learned, were party poopers who loved droning on about one thing—*at a time*—while my brain was busy connecting an inexhaustible flurry of seemingly unconnectable factors. There are no ideas I can't smoosh together. Munchausen syndrome by proxy, Ring Dings, and the native squashes of North America? Done.

In all art, patterns shift and become new patterns. If an artist doesn't shift, the viewer gets bored, unless the artist's aim is to defy expectations of shifting by shifting ever so slightly—like an Agnes Martin painting or a John Cage composition—or by not shifting at all, like Warhol's *Sleep*. Poets who don't shift or who "sneaky shift" are out there, but I'm here for the all-you-can-shift buffet. The murmuration of starlings. As essayist, author, cultural critic, and OG blogger Maria Popova said, "We have to be able to connect countless dots, to cross-pollinate ideas from a wealth of disciplines, to combine and recombine these pieces and build new castles."[1]

1 Maria Popova, "Networked Knowledge and Combinatorial Creativity," *The Marginalian*, August 1, 2011, https://www.themarginalian.org/2011/08/01/networked-knowledge-combinatorial-creativity/.

My new castles are everywhere, but few are inhabitable.

"You are *so wrong* about things sometimes!" a friend once marveled.

"I know! I'm like . . ." and made a "way out there" gesture.

". . . on another planet!" she hawed, then we hawed and hawed for hours.

People often assume that art is made by Individuals whose Brains are made of Diamonds. But what if you thought about art as a conversation between you and a ghost, or as ancestors chatting to the world through your mouth, or as a broadcast from a radio station at the center of the earth with you as its monophonic speaker? What if you were to imagine words and images floating around like pollen, looking for a hospitable spot to land?

I often refer to ghosts in my writing classes. "Did a ghost tell you to write that?" Nobody has ever replied, "What ghost?"

This is why there's no place I'd rather be than in a room full of poets.

When you read poetry, the areas of your brain processing that information—regions in the prefrontal cortex, medial temporal lobe, and posterior cingulate cortex—overlap with the areas involved in processing autobiographical memories and emotions that (your brain believes) are unique to you.[2] The more we read, the more the poem resembles us—like listening to a description of a stranger who turns out to be you. Surprise!

People with ADHD (sorry, I should've told you sooner, that's me) often struggle with episodic memory and executive functioning, the latter of which helps the neurotypical decide what actions to take both in the present and in the future to avoid repeating the past's

2 William O'Connor, "What Poetry Can Teach Us About the Brain," LinkedIn, March 21, 2023, https://www.linkedin.com/pulse/what-poetry-can-teach-us-brain-william-t-o-connor/.

mistakes.[3] How nice for them! For people with ADHD, though, after something happens, we may struggle to recall the order in which events occurred, details from the scene, and the emotions we felt at the time.

"I bought an ice cream maker! It's so awesome!" I texted my friend.

"Oh, honey. Don't you remember what happened to your last ice cream maker?"

"What?"

"You put it out on the curb."

"Because I was making too much ice cream?"

"Because you were making too much ice cream."

It's a good thing that poems don't need beginnings, middles, or ends. All I've ever needed was a good setup, which is what poems mostly are. As a kid, I would inhale the first one-third of a book and then, without a thought, abandon it. Now I see that my connection to art lies in what the piece *doesn't* do, which I'm compelled to imagine because of the uncanny things it *does* do.

In the final scene of Italo Calvino's *If on a Winter's Night a Traveler*, a stranger in a library says, "If a book truly interests me, I cannot follow it for more than a few lines before my mind, having seized on a thought that the text suggests to it, or a feeling, or a question, or an image, goes off on a tangent and springs from thought to thought, from image to image, in an itinerary of reasonings and fantasies that I feel the need to pursue to the end."[4]

If the end of the poem I'm writing surprises *me*, I feel I'm writing "right."

3 Russell Barkley, "What Is Executive Function? 7 Deficits Tied to ADHD," *ADDitude*, October 3, 2019, https://www.additudemag.com/7-executive-function-deficits-linked-to-adhd/.

4 Italo Calvino, *If on a Winter's Night a Traveler*, trans. William Weaver (Harcourt, 1981), 254.

For a long time, I wasn't sure I was a Poet. Even though all the poets I knew personally were freaks of various streaks, I thought the rest were detail-oriented, confident people with clean hands and average executive functioning. I will always be covered in the greasy sausage-smelling mist of Potentially and Dashed Expectations. I'll never be clean of it because I keep lathering myself into Incredible Hulk–level rages whenever I need to find a receipt or reset my password.

But sometimes Hulk is good. My high school guidance counselor once said, "If shoving an overstuffed trash bag into a shoebox were a sport, you'd be an Olympian." I'm not afraid of making mistakes. Heck, I make more mistakes before breakfast—on accident, on purpose, and in public—than most people make in a year. I treasure my mistakes because they don't need me to be right, and I make 'em fast—as many as possible—before some busybody pulls me over and scolds, "You're making a mistake, ma'am!"

"You mean, I *made* a mistake!" Sucker.

By the time I make a terrible decision, I've fallen madly in love with it, despite (because of?) the people yelling, "DON'T DO IT!" Somebody's got to throw a block of ice cream in a smoking pot of hot Crisco. Perhaps my brain can't tell the difference between alarm bells and doorbells. My love for bad decisions lasts as long as an awful hairstyle (e.g., a purple buzz cut): four months, which, coincidentally, is the same amount of time it takes to write a poem entirely based on terrible decisions, submit it, and get it published! The more terrible your decisions, the faster the poem will go to the press!

The first time I felt the speed at which poetry shifted was at a reading to celebrate the publication of *The Bird Catcher*, the collected poems of Marie Ponsot.

"Winter," Ponsot tolled in a voice as round and smooth as an egg.

My attention flared and—*poof!*—was gone, as usual. But then it was back, and I was listening to her paint the poem as it opened and opened. Every three or four words, a world bloomed, till the last line, where two worlds snuffed each other out. The speed at which her poem did this, using only ordinary words as fuel, felt entirely beyond words.[5] Though her steps from one end of the poem to the other seemed short, each was a lifetime. Maybe poems light up shapes that have been waiting to be seen.

*

In "Secrets of the Creative Brain," neurologist Nancy C. Andreasen uses an analogy involving kites, inventors, and engineers to compare generative thinkers and editorial thinkers. Inventors are like kites, moving in a million messy directions at once. Steady-handed engineers are the ones steering the kite with the string.[6] In my experience, people who encounter this analogy know which task their brain prefers, and very few people are equally good at both.

The more risks you take when you generate, the more of an ice-cold editor you will have to be later.[7] And I am not! Imagine opening a poem you wrote last week only to find it's a photograph of you from junior high school—and it's of the first time you got drunk, moreover, which is also the first time you asked a stranger to make out and promptly barfed on their shoes. That's 80% of my first drafts, so when I edit, I take my original intentions into the backyard and throw an in-

5 "Poetry, which, paradoxically, is not really a language art as we know fiction to be, is perhaps, as you suggest, more related to painting. But even more, perhaps silent film, because dreams, if not completely, are mainly wordless. The babyish subconscious doesn't know how to speak. It is the land of physical understandings. Its language is a language of images. Poetry is a physical art without a physical presence. . . ." Mark Tursi, "An Interview with Russell Edson," *Double Room*, no. 4 (Spring/Summer 2004), https://doubleroomjournal.com/issue_four/Russell_Edson.html.

6 Nancy C. Andreasen, "Secrets of the Creative Brain," *Atlantic Monthly*, July/August 2014, https://www.theatlantic.com/magazine/archive/2014/07/secrets-of-the-creative-brain/372299/.

7 If you, too, make more mistakes before breakfast than most people make in a year, let's repeat the Risk Takers' Oath! "Risk takers always take all the risks! / Not just the risks with happy endings! / That's not risk unless you have / average executive functioning, / which we don't, so we're risk takers!" Repeat 1,000 times.

visible ball as hard as I can into space while I cheer, "Go get it, girl!"—and she always does.

My subconscious tends to wipe out all my procedural memories of writing poems, and I used to marvel at how different my poems were from each other, as if I willed them into separate orbits—each a Möbius-strip universe of creation and collapse! Then my therapist suggested, "Maybe each poem's different because you don't remember how you wrote the last one. How you describe it sounds like you were in a trance state." Okay, that made a lot of sense. A new poem's not "I will do *this*!" It's "How did I do *what*?"

"Close your eyes and visualize. Are you in the house?" my new therapist asks. It's our second meeting, but I still have to write her name on the back of my hand with a Sharpie: "KATE." She sits across the room from me, watching me visualize myself standing in my childhood home—and maybe she's also mentally taking pictures of me, mentally drawing horns on my head in an app, and mentally texting them to her friends, "OMG, I HATE MY JOB!"

That last part was my rejection sensitivity dysphoria talking. Ninety-nine percent of children, adolescents, and adults with ADHD experience RSD, which begins when a person perceives rejection before they've even had a chance to be accepted or believes that they've failed at a task before they've even undertaken it.[8] This perception emotionally internalizes at a high intensity and manifests as long crying sessions, intrusive thoughts, psychological pain, and, sometimes, thoughts of suicide.[9]

8 William Dodson, MD, LF-APA, "How ADHD Ignites Rejection Sensitive Dysphoria," *ADDitude*, February 28, 2020, https://www.additudemag.com/rejection-sensitive-dysphoria-and-adhd/.

9 Nichole Currie, "What Is Rejection Sensitive Dysphoria, and Why Does It Impact People with ADHD?," The Pulse, WHYY, PBS, April 23, 2023, https://whyy.org/segments/what-is-rejection-sensitive-dysphoria-and-why-does-it-impact-people-with-adhd/.

"Mm," I grunt in reply. *You don't know me, Kate*, says my inside voice. Because I feel vulnerable with this new person, I've turned up all my apathy signals: I arrived twelve minutes late, feigning distractedness (it was easy), and made a haughty "hmph" sound as I theatrically turned off my phone. (In truth, I lost the charger—it's been out of juice for days.) Until I'm 100% certain Kate can handle my shame, I'll be 1,000% positive that she was sent by some sinister agency to find evidence of my humiliating mistakes. *Piece of cake, Kate: they're everywhere!*

"Breeeeeeathe," she hums, and I doooooooo. I like breathing as much as the next person, but it's so much breathier when someone *tells* me to breathe.

"Find the child," Kate nudges.

"Ung," I grunt, and float into the kitchen.

Here I am: ankle-deep in eggshells, spilled sugar, and butter wrappers, staring at black smoke billowing from a frying pan. I'm proud to see that I'm rocking my favorite outfit of all time: no pants and a 1970s grown man's sports shirt with a coveted ring-pull zip closure, stolen from my father's closet. I may have been wearing this shirt for days, floating around the playground and grocery store like a mauve-taupe terry-cloth jellyfish.

"What's she doing?" Kate asks.

I inhale a deep breath of depersonalization and exhale it over myself. The words that come to me are *sour*, *flabby*, and *vulnerable*. Suddenly, she/I, the egg-burning child, looks straight at me.

"Enh!" I gasp.

"What's happening?" Kate asks.

"Will you watch the omelet?" she/I asks, offering me the spatula, which I accept. "My song's on," she/I says, and zips out.

I find me in the living room, pretending to tap dance and singing along with a Jack in the Box commercial.

"Come as you like, come as you are, to Jack in the Boooooox . . ."

Her/my dancing is . . . interesting: enthusiastic, unpredictable, and less frightening than the smoldering space-out we had in the kitchen.

She/I pivots from heel-toes and shoulder rolls to floaty squid squats, karate kicks, and finger snaps, like if David Byrne and Jackie Chan performed the "Gee, Officer Krupke" number from *West Side Story*.

"You dance good," I say, and try to smile in a non-weird way.

Her/my brow is furrowed in concentration. "First I'll teach you how to dance, then we'll go get tacos."

Later, Kate asks if we were nervous.

I think about it. "Just me."

*

I'm unsure if this happened or if I dreamed it: somebody in my undergrad workshop was fired up about a W. S. Merwin poem he'd read. It was a dialogue between two little old ladies arguing about which cruise was better: Alaska or Hawaii. Their criteria were nearly identical *and* comically vague, which sounded like my kind of party.[10]

"What happens at the end?" I asked.

"*Nothing*," he scoffed, "it's a *poem*."

Nothing, indeed, though I loved the idea of Merwin talking in two voices so seemingly different from his own. Soon after, I wrote a poem in which an Earnest Ditz recalls a Snooty Norm telling her "all about a wonderful book she'd read" called *Mary Todd Lincoln*. Snooty Norm's recollections from the book are limited to hoop skirts, carriage rides, and grotesquely rich meals—more like a romantic novel than the biography of one of the most villainized First Ladies in US history, whom reporters nicknamed "the female wildcat." Snooty Norm seemed protective of her memories of the book, as if by having read it, she'd infused herself with fancy-pants-ness. Listening to Snooty Norm, the Ditz grows increasingly excited and begins to repeat the phrase "Mary Todd Lincoln" as if the syllables were caviar and champagne.

10 I've never been able to find this poem.

Suddenly, I felt bad for the Ditz—this wasn't a fair fight. How could I get her out of the poem, fast, and with a shred of dignity intact? Suddenly, the Ditz interrupted the Norm:

> "Did the book say anything about
> Mary Todd Lincoln chasing her husband
> around the White House with a butcher knife?"

The Snooty Norm started to talk and said, "Nnnnoooo."

What happened next in my head looked like this: The bus driver of the poem did a trust fall out the back and disappeared. Clogged energy fermenting in my body vaporized through my skin as clear, clean water. I was marveling at my permeability when a masked wrestler burst in out of nowhere, flipped the poem on its back, and Ditz's proud, final words shot out like grease through a goose:

> which doesn't make me
> different from anyone else
> named Mary Todd Lincoln.

I felt the poem tap out, which, to my workshop colleague, probably looked identical to nothing.

PROMPT: Tigers vs. Clouds

This prompt was inspired by three words Jim Galvin uttered in an undergraduate workshop: "Needs more tigers." Piqued by the evocative one-two punch of "more tigers," we demanded a thorough explanation. A poem, Jim said, is like one of those Chinese ink-wash paintings wherein the central figure, such as a tiger, or a detail of the central figure, such as a tiger's tongue, is rendered with hyper-clarity in juxtaposition to a less-detailed figure, such as a cloud.[11]

Any word can be a tiger or a cloud, depending on its surroundings. An old Polaroid of an empty parking lot lying on top of a pile of snow is a tiger. But laying it next to a guinea pig wearing a tiny sequined cowboy hat, it becomes a cloud. Because tigers require more description, a single tiger can be a two- or three-word phrase like "wet mitten" or "tan gummy bear."

An all-tiger poem in which every element "goes up to 11" in the detail department would be exhausting for a reader. Similarly, an all-cloud piece might struggle to hold a reader's attention, and while holding the reader's attention isn't the goal of every poet, it's my goal. I want to tap into the reader's dopamine-tastic reward center by way of surprise, but people can't be surprised if they're not paying attention because the poem lost them.

Let's say your reader feels pretty much oriented in the poem's first and second lines. Their reward center will be clanging like a ride at Coney Island, and they will follow your poem anywhere— from a little orientation drop-off at the volta to a *wtf is happening*

11 Jim was a master at describing abstract concepts using diction more often seen in small-town police blotter reports and auto repair manuals. It would usually go a little like this: "If this poem were a VW bus, and we had to drive it from Aurora to Lake Arrowhead, what would we need to put in the tank to get us there?" [silence] "Let's start with a title." This was extremely helpful because the language of literary theory bounces off me like a hail of Nerf darts.

tornado at the end. But if a reader feels disoriented primarily in the first line and then even more so further on, the reader's brain might wonder, "What's on TV?"

Shifting the reader's tiger-cloud focus across varying detail levels is one way to modulate the poem's situational tempo. Let's say you take four lines to describe the tiger's whiskers. Then, in one line (or maybe just a few words), you describe a rabbit that slipped into the yard where the tiger is taking a nap. Then, back to the tiger's tail for another four lines. More lines mean more information and more time for the reader to linger—thus, the tiger slows down, comes into focus. Especially in comparison to the one-line rabbit that zips by—a blurry blink. The steps below invite you to try writing with attention to these dynamics.

BONUS: While we were talking about the tiger, the rabbit ate all the lettuce in the garden. In boxing, this move is called a feint. "Look at my gorgeous tiger-esque right hand, so close to your head, swirling around and around and . . ." BOOM! goes the left hand. Try it.

TIP: Your tiger just is. Your cloud just is. Whatever you say they do, they do. No explanation or explication is necessary. Gravity is optional. You're the boss.

1. Think of a tiger-cloud pair. Your two words/phrases should be distinct in diction, rhythm, sound, or all three. The more distinct they are, the more surprising your results will be.
2. Write your tiger at the top of the left side of the paper and your cloud on the right. Example:

   [tiger:] melted gumdrop [cloud:] glare

3. Think of another tiger, but this time, choose one with some connection, direct or indirect, to your first tiger. In other words,

these tigers know each other. Write your second tiger under the first. Example:

[tiger 1:] melted gumdrop
[tiger 2:] blue Ring Pop

4. Think of another cloud using the same associative strategy as in Step 2. Write your second cloud under your first. Example:

[cloud 1:] glare
[cloud 2:] aura

5. Repeat the process in Steps 2 and 3 until you have five pairs of tigers and clouds, each associated with the pair above them.
6. Now you'll put them into a five-line poem, with each of the five lines containing one of the five pairs. Keep the lines as short as possible. Remember: No explanation or explication is necessary.
7. Now repeat Steps 2–5 to create five new pairs and five new lines. You may choose to connect the new words and lines to the earlier ones directly, indirectly, or not at all. Seeing your clouds and tigers in these new configurations will surprise your readers and turn on their reward centers. "Hoo boy! That cloud sure does get around!"
8. Don't look at the draft for at least a day as the generative writing go-go juice drains from your brain.
9. When you return to it, try to connect all ten lines to each other by adding or deleting some words at the front and back of the lines. The lines don't need to stay in the same order as you wrote them. Use as few connecting words as possible.
10. Remove all the words that don't need to be there.
11. Give the poem a very intimate, personal title, such as a name, an address, a date, an object, or an event from your past. Titles like this usually come to me when I wake up or when I'm getting out of the shower.

14

Finding Your Face

When Metaphor Becomes a Mask

EMILY STODDARD

For a long time, I believed that you don't actually need to "find" your voice as a writer. Your voice is always with you and can't be lost in the first place. This belief was shaped in part by mentors like Pat Schneider, who wrote: "You must trust your own voice. . . . Writers often ask me, 'How do I find my voice?' It is a sad question—as sad as if the question were, 'How do I find my face?'"[1]

But what if your voice has been transmitted through various masks for decades? What if your love of language isn't just a creative orientation to the world but also—maybe even more so—an unconscious coping mechanism?

In my mid-thirties, I found out that the restlessness, intensity, and impulsivity that stirred up my life (over and over again) were all aspects of unrecognized ADHD. Diagnosis felt like both an undoing and a homecoming: "Good news, you are indeed the alien you sensed you were. Bad news, you still have to be an alien on this planet. Good news, you now have language to find others like you. Bad news, you're going to use that new language to question everything."

1 Pat Schneider, *Writing Alone and with Others* (Oxford University Press, 2003), 93.

In my writing, this meant that I started questioning almost everything I thought I knew or believed about my voice. The more I learned about neurodivergent masking—a phenomenon of crafting a safer face for the world, a layer that shelters your intensities and makes you more appealing or legible to others—the more I wondered about the true purpose of the images, figurative language, and metaphors in my writing. Pat's words returned to me with a new, sharp edge: *It is a sad question—as sad as if the question were, "How do I find my face?"*

I began rereading essays and poems I had published, only to notice where I make caveats and cushion my voice. Only to spy whole passages where I was hedging my bets against being misunderstood. The first poem in my debut book is literally an incantation against being told you are "too much": "The trouble is everything calls to me. . . . Never say it is too much. Tell me it is only human—to wish for someone to believe in the myth of you."[2]

What does it mean to uncover yourself this way as a writer? And well after you've started publishing your work? What if my writing itself is the dressing room where I assemble and practice my masks?

What then?

Then maybe it's actually true, maybe I am actually asking: *How do I find my face?*

Is it a sad question? Or is it where I should begin now?

Growing up, one of my favorite rituals was going to the dime store with my grandmother, where she would let me pick out a small toy. I was always attracted to the paper dolls, with their array of clothing and the little tabs for dressing—easily torn, but also easily switched

2 Emily Stoddard, "More & More," in *Divination with a Human Heart Attached* (Game Over Books, 2023), 8–9.

out to imagine different lives for my flat characters. I could cast and recast the dolls into any story of my liking. I could make them dance or fly or run away from home.

I loved the orchestration of it. This kind of orchestration was how I was just beginning to make sense of myself and the little stranger-alien I felt I was. I could never just play pretend—I needed to be both absorbed in the scene and hovering outside of it, moving the parts to better understand them. If a storyline veered in a direction I didn't like or that might get confusing, I would sometimes announce, "Do-over! Do-over!" and reset. It was like trying to be the main character and the editor at the same time. It didn't earn me many friends, but it was probably the seed of my love of revision. In that sense, the orchestration felt true to me.

But in another sense, this orchestration had an element of vigilance to it. I felt a watchful hand nearby, always ready to moderate and adjust me in the same way I hovered above the paper dolls. An alert repositioning for an imagined audience, tracking each detail of self and story, trying to prevent misunderstanding at all costs. A paper doll is comfortable with this kind of hyper-attention. Unlike other children, the paper doll could tolerate my need to redo, reset, orchestrate another scenario. The wonderful yet risky thing about a mask is how it's such a willing collaborator. It can feel so agreeable, until you try to take it off. As I tabbed more layers over the flat shoulder of the doll, her eyes remained unblinking. We both knew better than to show how this work consumed us: the smile stayed open and receptive, in a premeditated display of happiness.

I needed to bring you to the paper dolls first, because that's how I always come to the page: I find an image for us to hold while I get into the work of composing myself.

This is not the first time I've tried to contort the paper dolls into a metaphor in my writing. I remembered them soon after I began sorting out what my neurodivergence means to my writing and my voice. When the memory arrived, it felt like a gift. It had that intuitive flash of This Must Mean Something. Maybe because I was questioning so much, the return of this childhood image felt like an offering of safety. (Maybe that's how I should have known it was another mask.)

Whatever the gift was supposed to mean, I pursued it like an assignment instead. The paper doll couldn't just be a memory—it would also be an idea, a concept, an image that I could fold myself into and use to hunt down something like revelation. I became especially attached to the language of "paper-dolling myself." It felt lyrical. It was a more beautiful way of saying the hard things I really needed to say. Behind the cover of the paper doll, I could write an essay that gestured toward my childhood, the early signs of trouble, the ways I navigated my family, the eventual collapse of a marriage, a career, a masked life. I believed that as long as the paper doll was the centerpiece, the story would tell itself.

It wasn't until another mentor, Jerald Walker, challenged me that I realized how far I was from the truth. It was all image and no story, he said. "Go try another version of this that never mentions a paper doll."

He might as well have said, "You've misplaced your face." He would have been right.

Now I'm here using the paper dolls again, but more selfishly and with impatience: I want to understand this impulse to shelter my voice in metaphor. And I also want to be done with the paper dolls. All that's left for them is to become the source of speculation in this essay. One last orchestrated hurrah, so I can no longer get away with stashing them in other essays, and then trying to stash myself inside of them. I have a hard time parting with metaphors, the paper dolls most of all. If I give them to you here, I can't take them back.

*

Do you ever feel sad for some of the masks you once wore? Do you ever wonder where they are now and what life they are having, on some parallel timeline? Especially the ones that felt true, until they fell apart? They were a part of you, in a way, weren't they? I want to talk more, hear more, know more about this kind of neurodivergent grief—the grief of the other timelines, the many metaphors lost and found on the way to a true voice—and how neurodivergent writers have to untangle it twice: first in their everyday lives, then again in the voice they compose on the page.

When I learned of my ADHD, my brother said, "You must feel so vindicated." Because I always knew I needed more answers. Because I always knew something felt wrong, or at least hidden. Because I tried. I really tried to get help. But vindicated—no. (Do you ever wish you didn't know the truth after all, because now it punctuates all the griefs and attempts along the way? Because it makes them that much more real and that much more unanswered? How can I feel vindicated when there are so many new questions to ask?)

Maybe I should stop asking sad questions.

After all, at face value, a mask is just another way of appearing in the world. At face value, metaphor is not inherently good or bad, helpful or harmful.

But I am here looking for my face, so I hesitate to take anything at face value now.

Instead, I find myself wondering whether my need to seek metaphor first—exhaustively and almost exclusively—is one of my most persistent forms of masking.

I wonder if this still serves my writing or if it only complicates the work of bringing out my true voice. Because rather than saying the thing directly and plainly, I shroud and symbolize my writing. At times, I decorate it. Not always realizing that in hugging so close to metaphor, I have distanced myself from what I really need to say.

Do I fear plainness in my writing?

Repulsed is the word I hear when I write that question.

It's true. Plainness repulses me.

I want to add caveats here immediately, in case you're confused by this interjection. I want to soften the riff. I want to tamp down any idea you have that I'm getting too passionate, too hyperbolic, too intense about this. Because if we were together now, you could have seen my nose squinch up and my hands flare in front of my body as I stepped back. You might have caught the sharp pitch of my voice when I blurted out: *Plainness repulses me*.

I know, I see it too: How plainly I just said that, and how unavoidable and clear the feeling was for having said it so plain. How the plainness became its own portal to meaning. But look how it leaves me standing out there—the naked thought, exposed. I can still feel it in my hands—the electricity of the blurt.

It would be much easier (safer, more familiar, more poetic) for me to conjure a strange bird for you here, or to point your gaze to a body of water and remind you how water takes on many forms and refuses to be just one thing, and even when you wade in the shoreline, your feet are mingling with something pulled up from the depths. Water refuses plainness. Here I am, pulling Lake Michigan over my face again—and if I haven't masked this well enough yet, just wait. Any moment now I'm going to start painting the unreachable and choppy horizon line for you (horizon lines being my favorite personal cliché), and this is how I will transmit my restlessness and my repulsion without ever showing you my face.

But I started with the plain truth this time, instead of starting with metaphor, and now I'm stuck with it. I'm not going to edit it out, for the sake of being honest with you. And that means I can't avoid how much clearer and more real it is to just say it: I fear plainness. Plainness exposes me.

*

(What if when you take off your masks you find out how plain and honest your face is? What if when you peel away your poetry and your metaphors, you discover your voice is stark, unadorned, but also unavoidable—not a symbol, but just you, penetrating each sentence? What if when you finally hear the true tone of your voice, it startles you in the best way?)

*

After the messy process with the paper dolls, I tried mapping other metaphors I've used in my writing over the years. I thought I could parse out which ones might be masks and which ones might reflect my true voice, and that this might tell me something about where my instincts end and overcompensation begins. I thought it could be a clarifying exercise. I thought it might help me feel the shape of my face, under the mask.

The trouble was how quickly my curiosity turned into self-skepticism, verging on self-surveillance. The hovering hand was eager for the chance to reappear, but now I was more aware of it, and it felt heavier. So many of my creative patterns and instinctive choices could also be sources of doubt: Is this true? Is this really me? How would I honestly show up in this moment, if I was unmasked and honoring how I'm wired?

This can be a slippery line of questioning for a neurodivergent writer, depending on where it falls in your process and how obsessively you pursue it. Invite these questions into your raw material and early drafts, and you could stay there forever. You could stop after every sentence and never let anything accumulate. Or you could bring these questions into the revision process too early and cut and tighten and prune yourself beyond recognition.

But I've had enough of editing and performing myself like that. I did not seek a diagnosis to find more ways to hyper-manage myself. I needed to figure out who I am so that I could free myself to show up in a steadier, more complete and honest way.

Here's what I've (roughly, tentatively) come to understand: There are metaphors that reveal, and there are metaphors that explain. When I enter the realm of explanation, a mask is likely in play.

Revelation feels like a portal. To me, it feels like the free-associating, riffing, constellating heart of ADHD. With my first book, most of the images arrived in dreams and then I followed them into the writing. For the most part, I did not know why they had shown up until many months into the project. I did not demand or prescribe meaning—the writing pulled out the meaning. Mostly I felt like I was listening, rather than writing. Now I try to stay open to (or at least curious about) that sensation whenever I write. When I'm listening, it's less likely that I'm working from a masked place.

Explanatory metaphors, on the other hand, feel more prescriptive and performative. This was my relationship with the paper doll. From the start it was a more conclusive metaphor, rather than an expansive one. I needed it to perform in a specific way, so it struggled to be generative. It would take many drafts before I realized that, but now I think that's an important tell of a metaphor-as-mask: it shows up with a job to do. It's committed to playing its role well. Sometimes too committed. This is part of what makes a mask so protective (and sometimes necessary) when navigating a neuro-normative world. But as a writer, this is limiting and even destructive to the work—instead of generating new possibilities, it smothers them.

This is not meant to be a harsh binary of good metaphor/bad metaphor. To me, it's a simple and loose organizing principle to start noticing when I lean on a metaphor as a mask, instead of following it into new (and hopefully truer) possibilities for my voice. It's a way of observing myself in the act of writing without becoming skeptical of myself.

*

Maybe it's true that I am asking, *How do I find my face?*

Maybe it's not true that it's a sad question.

When I listen with my constellation mind, the question becomes more divergent, curious, a space of possibility.

Suddenly I'm aware of how plain it is: *How do I find my face?*

I can't avoid it.

The question is not: *Why did I lose my face?*

Or even: *What does my face mean?*

Just: *How do I find it?*

There might be a thousand possible answers. I want to believe they might startle me in the best way.

PROMPT: Listening in Reverse

This prompt helps me remember that I can start working with a metaphor/potential mask in drafts *without having to know why* the metaphor/mask is showing up. There's something exhaustive and pathologizing about always having to interrogate the *why* to be able to move forward. How easy it is to convince myself that I'm "clarifying" my drafts, when in reality I'm only ruminating on them. This exercise could work with prose or poetry.

1. Return to a draft that feels stuck, stifled, or half-baked—even if you're not sure why it feels that way. Now pick a metaphor, a strong image, or a symbol that you notice recurring in the draft.
2. Working backward, from the end of your draft to the beginning, rewrite each paragraph or stanza without that metaphor, image, or symbol. I suggest beginning at the end for many reasons: to honor your spiral-brain and make this interesting; to free you from telling this story the way it's always been told; to find asides and overshares and ramblings that you might have ignored when you were putting the story in the "right order." If you feel stuck, worry less about crafting a beautiful explanation of what you mean and instead try a plain possibility to start your next sentence: "I am here to remember . . ." Repeat

this phrase as often as needed. Repetition like this is one of my favorite ways to get unstuck—it's a stimulus that can help you to keep writing, keep writing, keep writing.

3. When you reach the beginning of the draft, let the writing land wherever it lands without reviewing it immediately. I like to let the piece rest at least overnight. If new lines, fragments, or questions float into your mind while the piece is at rest, jot them down so you can incorporate them later, when you return to the piece.
4. To bring the revision to an intentional close, write down five potential titles for this piece, aiming to make each one weirder or more opinionated than the last. A rough title list like this celebrates where you've just traveled with the piece and can serve as a reminder for your next revision session. It's like a list of dreams the draft is having about itself as it awaits your return.

15

Waking, Sleeping, Dreaming

On Poetry and Getting Lost

CHLOE MARTINEZ

When I think about sitting down to write, I think about Blaise Cendrars's poem "Waking Up":

Waking Up

I'm naked
I've already taken my bath
I rub on some cologne
A sailboat is buffeted across my porthole
It's cold this morning
There's some fog
I straighten my papers
I set up a schedule
My days will be busy
I don't have a minute to lose
I write

—BLAISE CENDRARS, trans. Ron Padgett[1]

This poem seems to me to contain my ideal writing conditions: sensory excitement, freedom, order, time, simplicity, solitude, urgency. How

1 Blaise Cendrars, "Waking Up" from *Complete Poems* by Blaise Cendrars, translated and edited by Ron Padgett. Copyright © 1992 by Ron Padgett. Reprinted by permission of the University of California Press.

much solitude? The amount you have when you're in a cabin on a ship at sea. How much simplicity? So much simplicity that both clothing and punctuation are completely beside the point. No clutter, because how much stuff can you even have in a tiny ship cabin? This poem doesn't care about food or caffeine; its necessities are the scent of the cologne, the feel of the cold, damp air, a glimpse of a boat moving across a tiny field of vision. How urgent? "I don't have a minute to lose / I write."

The poem's title in French is "Réveil." Padgett's translation of the word, "waking up," feels perfect to me, but its more expansive meaning is helpful too: awakening or revival, as in the body or the mind coming alive again. No one actually wakes from sleep in this poem—that's already happened when the poem begins. The "waking up" referenced here, then, must be the experience of writing itself: the experience of being fully engaged and immersed, of accessing something utterly different from everyday life. The rest of the world becomes as incidental as "some fog" or a boat passing the window. The waking life is writing, and everything else might as well be a dream.

*

When I sit down to write, it's not at all like Cendrars's poem. I am not in a cabin on a ship at sea; I am on the couch, having dragged myself out of bed at 5 or 6 a.m. to get in an hour or two of writing before my kids wake up. I tiptoe across a floor strewn with toy dragons, trying not to step on a sharp wing. I do this because the early morning hours are when I can most often find that dream state out of which poems come. Later I will get to my office on the campus where I teach, and I might have some writing time between other work activities, but by then I'll be in the day, and things won't be so simple. There will be administrative tasks, meetings, prepping for and teaching classes, the rude interruptions of meals. I may go to look up the meaning of "*réveil*" and find that hours have passed and I'm late to pick up my kids from school. When I'm awake to everyday life, it's hard to recapture the dream that is writing a poem.

There are circumstances that may change for me in my writing life. What won't change is the fact that my brain is an ADHD brain, and I live perpetually in conditions that aren't designed for me. Despite my inability to accurately assess how much time it might take to do a task (or how many tasks I might be able to fit into the available time), deadlines and schedules continue, maddeningly, to exist. Despite my gift for hyperfocusing on what interests me (and doing that thing immediately), on any given day I need to do things that I don't find at all interesting or that aren't grabbing my attention just then. Despite my predilection for associative thinking, creative work, and constant variety, there's a lot that I must do in a fixed, predetermined, linear way, over and over again. Despite my inability to ignore birds and clouds and a kid biking by with his bike reared up on the back wheel like a horse, I sometimes need to talk with other people, which means I need to listen, ask questions, retain important details, and not constantly interrupt to say, "Oh, look at that kid on the bike! I think that bird is a dark-eyed junco, hang on, let me look it up!"

Poetry, on the other hand. Poetry and I were made for each other. Poetry is not productive. It doesn't happen on a schedule, and, assuming you're not in a class, no one is waiting for it. Poetry has no market value, no late fee, no annual review. You absolutely cannot write a good poem if you aren't interested in writing that poem; a poem happens only when the poet's interest shows up. I don't really agree with people who say poetry has *no* rules, but it can have as few or as many as you want. And whether you agree to rules or not, the many tiny engines driving a poem are engines not of law and order but of interest and impulse: music, disruption, juxtaposition, surprise, image. A poem needs the kid on the bike, and the dark-eyed junco, too. Wallace Stevens defined poetry as "the imagination pressing back against the pressure of reality,"[2] which feels exactly like what my brain is doing much of the time.

2 Wallace Stevens, *The Necessary Angel: Essays on Reality and the Imagination* (Vintage, 1942), 36.

And yet reality persists. As a dreamy person living in a structured world, negotiating between the two is a constant struggle. One of the reasons I love that Cendrars poem is that the only urgency it accepts is the urgency of writing: "I don't have a minute to lose / I write." This speaker in his little ship cabin isn't watching the clock to beat traffic. I, on the other hand, live between two California freeways (this is both metaphorically and literally true). Sometimes the pressure of everyday urgency makes it hard to find my way back to writing. Work-arounds such as my early morning writing sessions help, but my attention will always be a flighty thing, sometimes taking me deep into poetry and other times gone, an absent friend who won't call back. A taxi in a downpour during rush hour. I'm on the curb, soaked through, waving desperately.

*

It's not easy for me to share this, especially once my whirring brain begins to imagine possible readers: my students, my colleagues, people who have written me recommendation letters for stuff. That one person who, when I shared with a LISTSERV that I was working on a book project about writing and ADHD, wrote back, "Gosh, so many conditions, so little time! Sorry I can't help with this one. Good luck!" Nah, just kidding. That person is a jerk, and I don't care about their opinion. But I am nervous about the rest of you. I have spent years keeping the chaos pretty well covered up, for fear that someone might judge me as frivolous, unreliable, undisciplined, unprofessional, or whiny.

I'm sharing it now because the decision to own up to this mess—first to myself and then to others—has been one of the most liberating experiences of my writing life. Because ADHD doesn't actually make it difficult for me to write; it makes it difficult for me to do *everything else that writing requires*: completing ordinary tasks efficiently; shifting from one activity to another; filtering information to convey just what's needed in an email, class, or conversation; or scheduling something without giving the wrong date, time, or location. These processing tasks can overwhelm me and take up all my time. Sometimes they leave me an overstimulated mess at the end of the day, taking refuge in television. In turn, the hyperfocus of writing can temporarily make me forget time, space, and my own offspring, which is a blessing for my writing, a problem for the rest of my life.

*

I was diagnosed with ADHD in my late twenties. By then, I had managed to graduate from college with the help of a series of self-developed hacks and work-arounds, a lot of determination, a good support system, and strong writing and thinking abilities. But when I moved across the country and entered a PhD program in religious studies, I found that my old tricks were no longer enough. Suddenly I had to do very demanding academic work without much of a community, without the variety and flexibility of my undergrad coursework, and within a culture in which performing a kind of perfection was the norm.

I had entered the PhD program because I wanted to learn and teach about the religions of India (in particular, the role poetry plays in those religious traditions). I was totally unaware of the differences between college and graduate school. I soon discovered that my enthusiasm for the things I wanted to study was somewhat secondary to the competitive and performative aspects of academia. Everyone talked about the difficulty of what we were doing, but no one talked about feeling afraid they wouldn't measure up, their failures, or what they had to give up to do this weird thing. One woman in my cohort used to come into the grad student lounge and ask everyone what they got on a paper or exam, comparing scores publicly. It seemed clear to me that everyone was pretty unhappy—terrified of their advisors, of their inability to learn Sanskrit verb forms quickly enough, of being unable to make rent this month. It seemed as if being unhappy was expected, just part of what we were going through.

I was certainly one of those unhappy grad students, but along with the usual stresses of being in a PhD program, I was now watching all my ADHD hacks fail (though I didn't know yet that they were ADHD hacks). I was struggling to write papers without my best friends working alongside me through the late-night hours; to focus on extremely dense and specialized texts at the accelerated pace of as much as a full book per class each week; to bring my writing style into line with an increasingly inflexible set of scholarly conventions, many of which I actively disliked; to meet deadlines in a culture in which asking for extensions was even less acceptable than in college; to perform professionalism when I was constantly late, never prepared enough, losing confidence daily, and surrounded by people who seemed more polished than ever.

Even getting to class was a challenge. As an undergrad in New York City, I had walked everywhere and mastered public transit (how I loved the constant dopamine-generating puzzle and adventure of the NYC subway system). Arriving in California to begin my program, I quickly realized the bus system wasn't going to be very workable, and borrowed a little money from my grandparents to buy the cheapest working vehicle I could find: a fifteen-year-old Volvo station wagon (complete with an eight-track cassette player). I relearned how to drive stick shift, stalling out on every hill while people honked behind me. I regularly circled the maze of university parking lots, late for something, desperate for a spot that wasn't a mile away from my building. Misreading or ignoring signs about who could park where or running over my paid time, I got so many parking tickets that my car was "booted" more than once. I made some good friends in my program, none of whom seemed to be struggling the way I was. At some point during my first year, I sank into a serious depression and I thought about dropping out. The therapist who was saving me on a weekly basis finally suggested I get screened for ADHD.

Getting the diagnosis didn't solve any of my problems, but things made a little more sense after that. I realized that I had been working with a neurodivergent brain, which meant that I was at a significant advantage for some things, like creative problem-solving, associative thinking, deep research, and hyperfocus, while also at a disadvantage for others, like managing time and deadlines, working independently, and remembering to do necessary everyday tasks (paying a bill, finding my keys, eating when my body needed food). It explained why it took me multiple introductions to learn a new name, and why I often felt exhausted after trying to focus on long lectures or conversations with multiple people.

It also explained a lot about my love of poetry. "Poets speak inwardly," writes Craig Morgan Teicher, "talking into their minds and listening for their minds' responses."[3] I began to understand that the interior voice that was poetry, a voice that never minded if I spaced out or jumped to a new conversation, was not only suited to me but necessary for me. That perhaps I had always been drawn to the freedom of poetry as a refuge and respite from the struggle of daily existence in a neurotypical world. I considered the possibility that every time I'd been late to meet a friend or missed a deadline or forgotten a birthday or talked too much about something that excited me, it might *not* have been because I was a bad or lazy person.

I stayed in the PhD program, where I met my husband and got married. I wrote poems secretively, then took a year off to do an MFA in creative writing. Then a second MFA in poetry, low residency this time, concurrent with my dissertation work. Even though writing poems came much more easily to me than seminar papers, it didn't come easy. I turned in drafts and packets of work up to and beyond deadlines, despite my attempts to sit at my desk, like a private eye on a stakeout, until a poem appeared.

3 Craig Morgan Teicher, *We Begin in Gladness: How Poets Progress* (Graywolf, 2018), 4.

The kindness, though, of my teachers, sending me a gentle email nudge to ask if the work was coming soon—sometimes I come across those emails now, when searching for something else, and they make me cry. I felt horribly ashamed to have to ask my teachers, poets I absolutely idolized, for extensions, but I felt at least that they valued me and my work, and that they understood that people are complex and imperfect, which was very different from my experiences in the PhD program. At the end of one term, my cohort of MFA students at Boston University asked our teacher, Robert Pinsky, what his writing routine was like. Pinsky—a former US Poet Laureate and author of a stack of acclaimed books of poetry, prose, and translation—said something to the effect of "I usually write when I'm supposed to be doing something else." *Yes*, I thought.

After the MFAs, the PhD was still there, waiting for me. I was in my mid-thirties by that point, and my husband and I wanted to have a baby. For two graduate students, starting a family wasn't part of the recommended curriculum. A grad student friend of mine was told by a faculty member, *Every child you have is a book you won't write*. My friend did not listen to this advice, and neither did we. As a pregnant woman, I often felt strangely celebrated. People smiled at me and congratulated me on the street; strangers invaded my personal space, touching my belly and oversharing. My relatives were weirdly proud of me. Pregnancy was full of discomforts, but those, too, were recognized. People offered me their seats on the train, and my husband rubbed my feet, and I was given, in general, sympathy and help. For me it was an odd experience of rightness, of doing a kind of private work that was publicly marked as good, even sacred. I know that isn't everyone's experience; I was a straight, cis, married woman who hadn't had much difficulty conceiving, and my pregnancies were relatively uncomplicated ones. I was lucky in lots of ways.

When I finally transformed from pregnant lady to mother, everything changed. The pleasures of motherhood were visible from the outside: my daughter's chubby cheeks were admired, petted. Gifts arrived in the mail. But the cute parts of having a baby are public; the difficult parts are mostly private. The chaos and loneliness of new motherhood felt like something I couldn't talk about, shouldn't complain about—a struggle not unlike the ADHD masking I had been doing my whole life. My daughter's colic kept all three of us up every night, as my husband and I frantically tried to trick her into sleeping. We spent every night bouncing her, carrying her around, attempting to wrap her up in swaddle blankets that never seemed to stay put, and singing to her alongside various loud background noises that seemed to slightly soothe her—running water, fans, noise machines, pop music. Then we pretended to be functional humans during the day.

Other people seemed to be able to get their kids to sleep somehow. Friends, family, and an ever-growing stack of baby books advised us on various techniques, none of which worked. We had just moved and had no local support network: no one to witness and tell us it was okay, and no one to help. We once turned the car around halfway to the local mall because the baby was screaming so much. A crying baby or a melting-down toddler in public provoked embarrassment in me, and annoyance, disapproval, or useless unsolicited advice in others, so I did what I could to prevent those situations. I stayed home more. I wrote very few poems because when the baby napped, I needed to nap, too, or clean something, or stare into space.

When my daughter was old enough to leave her for longer stretches, I trudged to a tiny library cubicle to finish writing my dissertation, the clock of childcare or my husband's time away from his own work—we could hardly afford either—ticking away. I still remember the sensory experience of that cubicle: the dust, the way the light came in through the single tiny window, the particular smell of the old carpet, the weird chair. It was a space where the whole rest of my life was filtered out. It felt a little bit like punishment to go there day after day, but I wrote a whole dissertation that way. One cubicle day at a time.

Eventually, motherhood got easier, poetry came back to me, and life got more manageable. But looking back, I wonder if that brief experience of rightness, and the long wrongness of early motherhood that followed, set the stage for me to give up my notions of how I should be doing things, which is to say, to let me begin to do things in my own neurodivergent way. To understand that poetry was not merely a thing I liked; it was a whole world of experience that worked for me in ways that nothing else did. I don't think it's a coincidence that I started writing again in earnest while stroller-walking my second daughter around the neighborhood, sneaking in a draft while she (a better sleeper than her sister!) napped in the park. Nor is it accidental that those first poems in which I began to feel something happening again were about having a messy house, feeling like a mess of emotions, and making my own meandering, messy path through motherhood and writing. It was a relief to finally let that chaos show. Publishing many of those poems in magazines and then in my first book was an even bigger relief: it was really, truly okay to talk about these things. Eventually I put that work out in the world and was able to have conversations with other writers who shared these experiences. Sometimes I wonder how I survived for so long, thinking I was alone in these struggles.

*

One of the biggest challenges of ADHD is that the way our brains work doesn't always mesh with expectations of how we should do things. The result of that mismatch is that we can become experts at hiding our methods, our effort, and the many work-arounds we develop to do the things we want to do. We also spend a good deal of time feeling bad about that. It's a kind of double or even triple work: the thing we're doing, the extra things we need to do to accomplish that thing, and the cover-up, so that we can present to the world an acceptable narrative of ourselves and our work.

When I was in college, it seemed okay that I wrote most of my papers on pre-deadline all-nighters—everyone was doing that, and we did it together, in our dorm rooms and shared apartments and all-night library study spaces. But once I entered graduate school, I was expected to professionalize. I felt ashamed about how much I struggled to meet deadlines and to work without friends around. Now I know that body doubling (working with another person present), collaboration, and the urgency of approaching deadlines are all crucial ADHD hacks, and I employ them intentionally. I block off time closer to a deadline; I give myself grace and permission to be unproductive while I'm waiting for productivity to come; I collaborate, fidget, and change locations when I need to; sometimes when I'm stuck, I write lying stretched out on the floor, or standing up, or in a corner of a room where I've never sat before, or outside.

I do all this joyfully, knowing that I am finding ways to make the most of my neurodivergent brain instead of "doing it wrong." More and more, I mention my ADHD to colleagues or even to my students, not as a personal confession but as a passing comment. As if it were (though I know it still isn't) commonly shared, useful information, no different from telling someone you're left-handed. Now I think it's the shame, more than the ADHD itself, that takes a toll.

"When I had no roof I made / Audacity my roof," writes Pinsky in his great poem "Samurai Song."[4] I think about these lines all the time. When I gave up trying to write by forcing myself to sit at a desk on a schedule, I found that I sometimes enjoyed writing in a corner while something else was going on. When having children changed me from a night owl to an early riser, I discovered that writing in the predawn worked for me, not out of discipline but out of exigency. When I stopped searching for an "important" subject for my poems, I admitted that my own life was worthy of writing about and was a way to talk about bigger issues too, because the personal is always political. When I stopped carrying around a fancy notebook and chose a lightweight, small, temporary thing to write in, I wrote more easily. When submissions intimidated me, I made them into a game, sending out a packet of work to multiple magazines at once and celebrating each rejection, tracking them on an elaborate spreadsheet. When I had no institutional writing workshop, I made a workshop of my own with some friends—the best thing I've ever done for my writing. When I began to share my neurodivergent way of doing things with other people, first with a trusted few and eventually in front of a room full of people at a conference, I began to feel less ashamed, and less alone. *I'm that way too*, people said to me. I woke up to myself, and I rejoiced.

4 Robert Pinsky, "Samurai Song," in *Jersey Rain* (Farrar, Straus and Giroux, 2000), 3.

PROMPT: Customer Review

I like reading online product reviews. They're so intimate and so public, and they range from long, composed things to little dashed-off fragments of language. To mine reviews and shopping sites for something so unmarketable, so *unproductive*, as poetry seems to me like a tiny act of anti-capitalism, as well as a sidelong, nontraditional, very ADHD approach to poetic inspiration.

A poem of mine called "The God Structure" arose out of reading product reviews. I happened to read, in a review of a bra, "It has a god structure, I hope it will resist a long time." This odd sentence, with its typo and its somewhat non-standard use of "resist," sparked something for me. At the time I was processing a dear friend's recent sharing of his terminal medical diagnosis with me. The sentence from the review seemed to chime with everything I was feeling, and the poem came to me very quickly, with many of its final pieces intact. Retrospectively, I can see that the typo in the review was calling out to me as a textual stand-in for the slight difference in a cell or genetic code that can shape or destroy a life. The distance provided by looking at language that is not my own gave me access to what I needed to say.

1. Go to the shopping website of your choice and find an interesting bit of language in the customer reviews section, or maybe in a product description. Look for language that jumps out as awkward or confusing, or else as especially clear and evocative. Keep it short—a few words or a sentence is enough.
2. Now think about the thing that language is attached to. Consider why you might be drawn to or surprised by it, or how a similar item may figure in your life.

3. Freewrite using your chosen bit of language (and perhaps the item itself). You could do this however you want, but here are a few options:
   - Decide where the phrase goes in your piece, then write around/from/toward it.
   - Use it as a word bank (use all the words, but do something new with them).
   - Use it as an epigraph.
   - In a poem, use each word at the beginning of each line in order (sort of an acrostic), or at the end of each line in order (a take on a golden shovel). In prose, you could do the same thing with sentences or paragraphs instead of lines.

4. Extra points if the poem/prose also includes the following:
   - something constructed
   - something that grows
   - something you said in conversation that makes you uncomfortable

5. Consider whether that item you've chosen is related in any way to what you're writing about. Is the garden hose from which you've grabbed some text connected to drought (emotional or ecological), or to some kind of tangled problem you're trying to solve, or to a need to nurture something new? As you write or later, as you revise, consider whether that underlying concern is there in the piece, and whether it could be made more visible in any way.

Afterword: On Being Neurospicy and Everything Else

An ADHD Conversation with David Kessler

David Kessler is a practicing therapist, nationally recognized speaker, and ADHD advocate. He is the cofounder and clinical director of the Willow Center for Integrative Health in Chicago. He is also the cohost, with Isabelle Richards, of the podcast *Something Shiny*, in which "two therapists with ADHD help you build a shiny new relationship with your ADHD." The podcast takes down barriers to access for its listeners, offering clear explanations of concepts from neuroscience and psychology, in-depth conversations about the joys and challenges of this neurotype, and unexpected delights, such as explaining the different types of ADHD through the metaphor of buying a new printer. Toward the end of the editing process for this book, we sat down with David to get a therapist's perspective on ADHD and the creative life. Here's what happened.

On choosing what to wear for the interview

David Kessler (DK): Hello!

Chloe Martinez (CM): Hi!

Lisa Van Orman Hadley (LVH): Hi! Oh, I love your shirt!

[David is wearing a shirt that reads NEUROSPICY over an outline of a brain.]

DK: Yeah, I was like, what do I wear? Oh my god—I know exactly what I can wear.

On nonlinearity

DK: I'm just so excited to do this, and I love the idea of this book. I'm giving you full permission to rearrange any of this information in a linear way to make it make more sense.

[Note from Chloe and Lisa: We *did* rearrange much of the information in this conversation, but we did it in a very nonlinear way, because that made the most sense to us.]

On renaming ADHD and the idea of it being a disability

DK: If I could hit a button and rename ADHD right now, I would call it "attention variability."[1] I would get rid of the entire idea of it being a disability.

I was diagnosed as having a learning disability at a very young age, third grade. I struggled in school—had behavior problems, didn't get good grades, eventually got kicked out of high school. And then I was diagnosed with ADHD in college. When I first learned about ADHD, I learned about it as a disorder. It was a broken part of me that I had to compensate for.

So I first want to say that ADHD is *not* a learning disability per se. But it *can* be. ADHD differences are neurological differences.[2] We have a different kind of brain—it's not pathology, not necessarily dysfunction, not necessarily disability. I prefer the term "learning differences," but learning disabilities in schools are based on students' needs and struggles. So if somebody evidences that they really struggle in school, or that they need a lot

1 Callie M. Ginapp et al., "'Dysregulated Not Deficit': A Qualitative Study on Symptomatology of ADHD in Young Adults," *PLOS One* 18, no. 10 (October 12, 2023), https://doi.org/10.1371/journal.pone.0292721.

2 Yannis Paloyelis et al., "Functional MRI in ADHD: A Systematic Literature Review," *Expert Review of Neurotherapeutics* 7, no. 10 (2007), 1337–56, https://doi.org/10.1586/14737175.7.10.1337.

of help, or that accommodations are needed, that's when ADHD becomes a learning disability. The belief that an academic system is a level playing field is the largest bunch of malarkey I've ever seen. Your self-esteem is deeply damaged when you think it's a level playing field. You try to do everything the same as everyone else, and then you judge yourself for failing. It's like "Why can't I move my feet here? Everyone else is dancing!" If we treat learning differences as a problem that students have to solve on their own, it can put them at a major disadvantage. But if we normalize accommodating differences, that disadvantage can go away.

The three ingredients for the success of a person with ADHD or learning differences are self-esteem, advocacy, and metacognition. Self-esteem is not the belief that you're the best person in the world; it's just the belief that you can survive. It comes from repeated exposure. If you avoid things that make you uncomfortable, that's fine, but you're not building self-esteem in those areas. Advocacy is asking for the accommodations you need, and metacognition is knowing *why* those accommodations help you. That last piece is so important. When you understand that you need a certain kind of light to work optimally, you can look around at your space and notice, "Oh, this lighting is a problem for me." If you don't have that awareness, you might think, "I don't know what's wrong with this place. I just know that it sucks, and I gotta get out of here." Knowing what you need and why is a form of self-regulation. It helps you better understand how you react to the world. You can expect more consistency that way, rather than hoping that the best version of you will just magically show up.

On people who help you find something shiny in yourself

DK: When I was first coming into my adult self, I was introduced to three learning difference advocates from the mentoring program Eye to Eye—LeDerick Horne, Marcus Soutra, and David Flink—who helped reshape my perspective and understand that maybe the deficiency isn't with who I am, but with who I thought I was supposed to be.[3] I was trying to design a perfect mask to look neurotypical, and trying to have needs that were aligned with neurotypical people. It took a lot of energy for me to do that, because that's not how I naturally learn or acquire information, and that made me think that I wasn't good at acquiring information. Once I was exposed to the fact that there are lots of ways to learn, that's when I stopped masking as much.

After I was introduced to Eye to Eye (now called the Neurodiversity Alliance), I started talking about ADHD as much as I could. I felt that there needed to be a different voice, someone from within the ADHD community talking about ADHD in a nonbiased, non-pejorative way. The podcast was a way to make those kinds of conversations about ADHD accessible to a wider audience. It is a joint venture with Isabelle Richards, a therapist with ADHD. Isabelle is wickedly smart, and she's a really fun person to do stuff with. Her creativity is just unmatched. When we were brainstorming names for the podcast, Isabelle started talking about something shiny being the thing that distracts us, but our difference is also a positive part of who we are, how we shine. And we realized *Something Shiny* was the perfect name for the podcast.

On intersectionality

DK: We often don't talk about the fact that there are major cultural factors in how we think about learning differently and neuro-

3 Eye to Eye (https://eyetoeyenational.org/) is a national mentoring program that pairs college and high school students with learning differences and/or ADHD with similarly labeled middle-school students.

divergence.[4] Misogyny, racism, and systemic racism have shaped the way people have viewed ADHD. Women are judged more harshly for struggles with organization and managing a household, or for things like forgetting to bring cookies to your kid's school event. If you're Black, being late is judged as laziness, and being hyperactive can be seen as aggression. In these ways, the experiences of neurodivergent women as well as LGBTQ and BIPOC neurodivergent experiences are systemically invalidated, underdiagnosed, and underserved. These layers of experience and marginalization are cultural and need to be unwound piece by piece. That can only happen by honoring what these experiences are like for each of us.

On honoring your own recipe for creativity

DK: I think there's a romantic notion around *productivity* that gets in the way of *creativity*. People often romanticize what being productive looks like or what "work" looks like, and we don't validate the different ways we play with creativity. So, for example, someone might say to me, "I'm a very disorganized person." And then I'll say, "Okay. But you just threw a big party. How did you do that?" And they'll say, "Oh, I'm just really good at networking. I called all my friends and outsourced all the different tasks. They did all the work." In this moment, the person is invalidating all their skills, all the conversations they had, how they worked with all these different people.

When we look at life like that, we miss recipes for creativity. Are you telling stories? Are you making things up? Are you researching stuff? Are you having debates with people that further

4 Benjamin Zablotsky and Josephine M. Alford, "Racial and Ethnic Differences in the Prevalence of Attention-Deficit/Hyperactivity Disorder and Learning Disabilities Among US Children Aged 3–17 Years," NCHS Data Brief No. 358 (March 2020), https://www.cdc.gov/nchs/products/databriefs/db358.htm.

an idea you're going to write about? Maybe we invalidate those things because our way doesn't look like a traditional image of productivity.

Honor the recipe that makes you successful, not the recipe that somebody tells you will make you successful. Somebody might say, "Your writing needs to be a practice. Sit down every day for one hour and write." But a lot of folks with ADHD will find themselves working really late at night or really early in the morning. Some people need to be in a noisy coffee shop. Some people need to be in a place with no noise.

If you've seen one person with ADHD, you've seen *one person with ADHD*. We don't all need the same accommodations, but knowing which ones exist and finding environments that naturally shut out distractions for you are parts of the recipe.

On motivation

DK: A lot of interventions meant to inspire work actually destroy intrinsic motivation. There was this study where people were put alone in a room with a puzzle and told to solve it as many times as they could in eight minutes.[5] Half of the people were told that they would get $1 every time they completed the puzzle. The other half were not offered a reward. Eight minutes later, the researcher came back and told the people who were promised money, "We're going to review the footage now, so we can count how many times you solved the puzzle. We'll come back in eight minutes with your money." The other group was just told, "We're going to review the footage now, and we'll be back in eight min-

5 Kira Warje, "Why Do We Lose Interest in an Activity Once We Are Rewarded for It?" The Decision Lab, https://thedecisionlab.com/biases/overjustification-effect; Delia O'Hara, "The Intrinsic Motivation of Richard Ryan and Edward Deci," American Psychological Association, 2017, https://www.apa.org/members/content/intrinsic-motivation.

utes to tell you how many times you solved the puzzle." What they were really testing for was who kept playing with the toy. They found that the people who were promised payment stopped doing the puzzle once the monetary incentive was removed. But the people who weren't going to get paid kept solving the puzzle. Because otherwise they would sit there and be bored, right? The moment we start putting value on things, we change our motivation from internal to external.[6] And I think that so many writing systems around accountability play into that dynamic and aren't always successful. [You can find a list of David's favorite strategies and accommodations that *are* successful at the end of this interview.]

On dopamine and risk

DK: I think that there's a piece of creativity that needs to sit in a risky place, because creative work is uncharted territory. And people with ADHD are often drawn to risk.[7] That's because ADHD comes with a dopamine deficiency. Visualize a thimble: that represents how much dopamine most people need. The moment that thimble is full, a neurotypical person is satiated and can say, "Ah, I have watched enough TV" or "I have had enough chocolate." With an ADHD person, we replace the thimble with a pint glass. That same amount of dopamine never fills that pint glass, and the ADHD person never feels satiated; we are perpetually dopamine-starved. Different things elicit dopamine: the blue photons in screens, excitement of different kinds, and risk. The whole time you're in a risky situation, your brain has access to dopamine,

6 This reminded Lisa of Lewis Hyde's *The Gift: Creativity and the Artist in the Modern World* (Vintage Books, 2006).

7 Yehuda Pollak et al., "Risk-Taking Behavior in Attention Deficit/Hyperactivity Disorder (ADHD): A Review of Potential Underlying Mechanisms and of Interventions," *Current Psychiatry Reports* 21, no. 33 (March 22, 2019), https://doi.org/10.1007/s11920-019-1019-y.

and so an ADHD person is naturally reinforced to be a little bit of a line stepper.

Now, that's not necessarily about dangerous behavior. Let's think about risk in a very ADHD way. It's going to take thirty minutes to get to the airport, so I'm going to leave thirty minutes before my flight. That's risky, right? Because if I get stuck in traffic, I could be late and miss my flight. But if I'm lucky, I can get there on time. Whether I make it or not, I'm getting dopamine the whole time.

CM: This idea that ADHD people actually have a predilection for risk is so interesting to me. It's true, to be a creative person is to want to take risks all the time! I definitely see that when I offer creative assignments to students. Some of them will say, "Tell me how to do it." But some of them will just try it out. That's creativity: being excited to attempt the new thing, the unknown.

LVH: In my experience, writers with ADHD are more likely to write things that are experimental. They seem more willing to play around with form, chronology, genre, voice, et cetera. Chloe and I had an inkling that this was the case when we requested essays for this collection, and as the submissions started to come in, all our suspicions about ADHD writers, risk-taking, and innovation were confirmed.

DK: Yes! We're more prone to take both healthy and unhealthy risks, and that can really work in our favor as creative people. We also think differently. Our brains are supposed to do this thing called pruning, which cleans up our neurological connections, just the way you prune a plant. Well, ADHD brains don't do nearly as much pruning. So we have these incredibly complicated neurological nets, which help us to think and remember and reason in associative and nonlinear ways.

On creating on/off conditions

DK: I have a high degree of vulnerability to environmental differences, so I create on/off conditions to make a distinction for myself between work and play. I have specific things that I do for play, and very different things that I do for work. As a therapist, I have to write a note for every client I see; I also often work from home, and tend to want to get up and do something else right after I finish a session. So I have special headphones that I wear only for work, and I have a rule that I can't take them off until I've done all my notes for the day. There'll be times when I'm downstairs taking a short break and my partner will ask, "Why do you still have your headset on?" And I'll say, "I gotta go back and finish the notes." Once I've finished everything, I can take them off.

LVH: I'm thinking about Mr. Rogers and how he changes his shoes and puts a different sweater on to mark the start or finish of the workday. Or how the train in that show travels to the land of make-believe. When we watch the train go around the corner, we know that we're going to a new place now, where different kinds of things happen.

CM: This is interesting for writers, right? Because we often write at home and have a lot of control over our own schedules, and so the work day and work environment that would create all of those conditions and triggers and boundaries for us, writers often have to make them ourselves.

DK: With the writing experience, I would ask, "When did you have your great long sessions? When did it feel really great, and what did you have around you?" Those are probably things that you needed in your "on" condition. And that place where you tried to work and it didn't work? That's an "off" condition. Focusing on what works helps you create the conditions you need to succeed.

On boredom

DK: Being bored is uncomfortable, but it's actually an incredibly important thing for our brains. It's when we have ideas and process experiences. There's something called an ADHD stupor. So, for example, you're putting on your socks and all of a sudden you kind of stare off for a long time, not really thinking about anything, and then you snap back into putting on your socks. Because of our perception of time, people with ADHD experience more of these moments of nothingness than a neurotypical person does, and those moments can also lead us into thinking and dreaming. So much dreaming happens for people with ADHD. Dreaming provides a refuge, a place of safety, which is incredibly important for creativity. When we're experiencing a lot of boredom, really wonderful ideas can emerge.

LVH: The bulk of my writing is done during those moments of stupor or daydreaming—during the thinking and the ruminating that happens before the physical act of writing begins. And I wonder whether we sometimes don't allow ourselves enough time to dream, to build in time to just sit with our thoughts without the pressure to produce words on a page, instead of acknowledging that what we're producing in those moments in between writing is intangible but incredibly valuable.

DK: You need time to stew. When someone asks, "What did you do today?" it's very easy for us to think, "I did nothing all day." But what if you sat all day thinking about your book and instead you responded, "I worked on my book all day." That would also be honest. I want people to start validating that it doesn't have to look a certain way to count.

On finishing something when it feels like you're folding socks forever

LVH: Right before this interview, I was on a walk with my son. He's twelve and has ADHD, and he said, "I wish I could just stick with one project and make it really good." He's a coder and he'll start all these amazing projects, but then he'll get bored, and instead of finishing, he'll just start a new one. So he has maybe one hundred projects he has started and not finished. And I'm wondering, for writers, how can we sustain interest over the course of a project, especially when we're writing an entire book? How do we actually finish? Do you have any ideas about that?

DK: Oh my god, I have so many! The dam is fracturing, get ready [laughs]. Where do I start? Okay. So when we're talking about big projects, typically the parts that are hardest are the finishing details. When we first have a creative idea, it's exciting, but once it's framed out and it's time to fill in the details, those are the least rewarding, least dangerous, most mundane parts. For an ADHD person, that's like folding socks forever. And I think this is a moment where a difficulty can turn into a self-esteem-injuring thing: "I'm a bad person because I don't finish things."

Instead of blaming ourselves, we should find accommodations that work for us. For example, "I need to work with other people" or "I need body doubles" or "I could use a person who likes to take over the finishing touches." There's a whole other group of people, many of whom also have ADHD, who love doing those final tasks and hate the beginning of a project. If those people work together, they accommodate each other.

LVH: I think that Chloe is one of these "finishing touches" people! So many times while working on this book, I lost steam or got overwhelmed or didn't know where to go next, and Chloe jumped in and worked her magic to tidy up the remaining details like Mary Poppins snapping her fingers.

CM: In turn, I've often been overwhelmed by the blank page, and Lisa often took a first step that made things feel more manageable. Collaboration—specifically with Lisa—has become my favorite ADHD hack.

On guilt, shame, and turning the procrastination nightmare train into a compassion train

DK: If we're ashamed of something, we're not going to talk about it, which is one reason why some people don't tell other people they have ADHD. We tell ourselves things like "If I had done this work earlier I wouldn't be feeling like this. If I cared more and was a better person, I would have done this two weeks ago!" And I think that if we flip those things into compassion and gratitude—I know that sounds so fluffy, but if we actually do that stuff, it can really change the way our nervous system responds to things. Subtle compassion statements can make a real difference: "You didn't do anything wrong. This sucks but it's going to get better."

That whole awful nightmare train around procrastination when I was growing up? Now it's a train of compassion: "Of *course* you had to wait until the last minute to do this thing! What do you need for the next twenty-four hours? Do you have enough coffee? Do you have those snacks that you really want? Did you order pizza?"

CM: When Lisa proposed doing a panel on ADHD at a writers' conference, I thought, "Okay, well, maybe it'll just get rejected. I'm not going to think about the reality of having to stand in front of a room full of people and talk about this." And then it was accepted, and we had the panel and it was amazing. That was a really important turning point for me in thinking about what it would mean to talk about this thing in public. It *does* mean you actually have to really actively give up shame and guilt. I'm so grateful that we did it and that it's turned into this bigger, more public conversation for us.

DK: I recently attended a conference on neurodiversity. There were fidgets on every table, spaces to get up and move around, snacks. When you are surrounded by other neurodivergent people, the accommodations are already there. All of a sudden things are a little bit easier. When I say, "It was such a win, I got there with thirty seconds left," to someone who is neurodivergent, they understand. When I talk about organizing things in piles, or how hard it is to do boring tasks, or wanting to take a peek at danger, there is a cultural resonance, a shared experience among neurodivergent people. And when we deny that we have that culture, we surrender to ableism. I think the more we try to make ourselves look like other people, the more we are surrendering parts of ourselves that shouldn't be surrendered. When we hide these parts of ourselves, we miss joining the culture. But when we put ourselves out there and find more people like us, we can start building a community of people who think differently.

Additional Writing Ideas and Accommodations from David Kessler

- *Change your device screen to white text on a black background.* When you look at a white background on a screen, the blue photons trick your brain into believing it's looking at the sun. The brain produces dopamine in response, which ADHD people in particular crave. Changing the text to white allows you to put all that evocative dopamine power into the words instead of wasting it on the background. It also lessens the roller coaster of dopamine exposure and withdrawal—the thing that makes it hard for us to look up from our devices.[8]
- *Narrow the width of your digital page.* The longer the line, the greater the possibility of an eye-tracking error, especially if you have ADHD. That means you will skip and read the line below or above, and that won't make sense, and then you have to read the line again. That experience is punitive—it makes reading harder. People often naturally accommodate this by holding their hand under the line, or by highlighting the part they're reading so their eyes won't skip.
- *Use AI to outline and break down tasks.* I don't always love AI, but it can be a really helpful tool for ADHD folks. The *kinds* of

8 Ellen Littman, "Never Enough? Why ADHD Brains Crave Stimulation," *ADDitude*, August 21, 2024, https://www.additudemag.com/brain-stimulation-and-adhd-cravings-dependency-and-regulation/; C. M. Rogers et al., "Color Contrast: Research," National Center on Educational Outcomes Accommodations Toolkit #25a (2022), https://publications.ici.umn.edu/nceo/accommodations-toolkit/color-contrast-research.

directions we give the AI are really important. So, instead of saying, hypothetically, "Finish my book for me," you could say, "Create an outline with these six characters meeting in a town, in this part of the world, with no trees, written for a fifth grader," and then it will create that outline for you. It can give you a starting point to then modify and do anything you want with. An app called Goblin Tools uses AI to break down any task into subtasks, which ADHD folks often have trouble doing on their own.

- *Use a digital timer or a visual timer.* [See "Selected Resources" for some options.]
- *Take advantage of apps.* There are apps that let you schedule text messages to send at specific times and dates in the future. So if you want to impulsively text somebody at 2:00 a.m. but know you shouldn't write to them in the middle of the night, you can set the text to be delivered at 8:30 a.m. so you can clear the thought out of your mind. Email also generally has a "schedule send" feature, so you can write when you need to and send later. Voice-to-text is really helpful for some people. Organization apps like Evernote let people connect different digital objects and save them together so all their notes are in one place.
- *Learn to ask questions.* Many neurodivergent people are scared to ask questions because they think they should already have the answers. When you're around people who make you afraid to ask questions, that's masking, and it makes for a disconnecting, sterile, marginalizing experience. But asking questions keeps us engaged and allows us to pay better attention. We need to find people and create environments that allow us to be curious and inquisitive.

Acknowledgments

We want to thank our editor, David B. Olsen, who saw a need for this book and trusted us to put it together. His generous feedback, keen editorial eye, and humor have made this process a joy and an affirmation for us. This book would not exist without him.

Thanks to everyone else at the University of Chicago Press who helped make this book a reality, particularly Matt Lang for handling the contributor contracts, Erin DeWitt for eagle-eyed copyediting and fact-checking, and the book designer Rae Ganci Hammers for her thoughtfulness around making the font and formatting accessible to an ADHD audience.

We are grateful to our contributors for their brilliant writing and for their graciousness throughout the editorial process; to David Kessler, for sharing his expertise with us; and to Rebecca Makkai, whose foreword is the perfect entry point into this book.

Thanks to the Association of Writers & Writing Programs for giving us the space, at the 2023 AWP Conference, to begin a public conversation about writing and ADHD. Thanks to our wonderful co-panelists: Tricia Caspers, Denise Delgado, and Daniel Jenkins. Enormous thanks to the audience of writers who showed up that day, making us see what an important conversation this was.

Lisa is grateful to Lars and Maud, whose excitement about their twin ADHD diagnoses helped her see all the bright parts of her own, and Dan, for his neurodivergent companionship and excellent jokes.

Their love and support are everything. She thanks her "Write or Dies"—Rachel Rueckert, Katie Rich, Kim Ence, and Barbara Brown—for reading many different versions of her essay and making it infinitely better each time; her psychiatrist, Allyce K. Jones, for her ever-expanding knowledge of and commitment to women with ADHD; her therapist, Abby Zeveloff, whose compassion and insights continue to be a source of comfort and growth; her ADHD meds, without which this book probably would have taken twice as long to finish; all the friends and family members who cheered on this project; her cat, Woodchip, the snuggliest writing companion; and the teachers who trusted her to do the work her own way. She is grateful to her dad, Bob Van Orman, and to her father-in-law, Paul Hadley, who both passed away while this book was being written. And most of all, she is grateful to Chloe, who single-handedly turned her from a skeptic into a believer in group projects. Thank you for your wit, intelligence, trust, instincts, compassion, hard work, body doubling, and magic making and for demonstrating that our ADHD way of doing things is not just valid but beautiful.

Chloe would like to thank Regan Huff for her sage advice early on, as well as the many other friends, colleagues, and family members who listened and offered encouragement, in particular, Julia Cheiffetz, Megan Davidson, Caribbean Fragoza, Kate Hollander, Lili Ibara, Lina Patel, Cynthia Prochaska, Nora Martinez Proctor, Prageeta Sharma, and Chrissy Crockett Sharp. Chloe is forever indebted to Jeanne Stanford, who suggested, so long ago, that she have an ADHD screening, and to Nayeli Corona-Zitman, whose care and insight have made all the difference. Deepest gratitude to her husband, Jamel Velji, for unflagging support and careful reading of drafts, and to Amina and Saafia, for being themselves. Finally, she thanks Lisa for diving into this project so enthusiastically, for understanding that the sidetracks were part of the process, and for making this collaboration the happy revelation that it has been from start to finish.

Chloe gratefully acknowledges Claremont McKenna College, in particular the Department of Religious Studies, the Center for Writing and Public Discourse, and the Gould Center for the Humanities, for support that made her work on this book possible.

Selected Resources for ADHD and Writing

Books

Davis, KC. *How to Keep House While Drowning: A Gentle Approach to Cleaning and Organizing*. Simon & Schuster, 2022.

Hallowell, Edward M. *ADHD Explained: Your Tool Kit to Understanding and Thriving*. DK, 2023.

Holderness, Penn, and Kim Holderness. *ADHD Is Awesome: A Guide to (Mostly) Thriving with ADHD*. Harper Horizon, 2024.

Huey, Amorak, and W. Todd Kaneko. *Poetry: A Writer's Guide and Anthology*. 2nd ed. Bloomsbury, 2024.

Ladau, Emily. *Demystifying Disability: What to Know, What to Say, and How to Be an Ally*. Ten Speed Press, 2021.

McCabe, Jessica. *How to ADHD: An Insider's Guide to Working with Your Brain (Not Against It)*. Rodale, 2024.

McConnell, Marty. *A Gathering of Voices: Creating a Community-Based Poetry Workshop*. YesYes Books, 2018.

Moss, Adam. *The Work of Art*. Penguin, 2024.

Otsuka, Tracy. *ADHD for Smart Ass Women*. HarperCollins, 2023.

Piepzna-Samarasinha, Leah Lakshmi. *Care Work: Dreaming Disability Justice*. Arsenal Pulp Press, 2018.

Salesses, Matthew. *Craft in the Real World: Rethinking Fiction Writing and Workshopping*. Catapult, 2021.

Silberman, Steve. *NeuroTribes: The Legacy of Autism and the Future of Neurodiversity*. Avery, 2016.

Terry, Philip, ed. *The Penguin Book of Oulipo: Queneau, Perec, Calvino and the Adventure of Form*. Penguin, 2020.

Wong, Alice, ed. *Disability Visibility: First-Person Stories from the Twenty-First Century*. Vintage, 2020.

Websites/Organizations

ADDitude (https://www.additudemag.com). Free online articles and resources related to ADHD.

CHADD (https://chadd.org). An organization offering information, advocacy, and support for people affected by ADHD.

Disability Matters (https://rjionline.org/news/a-toolkit-for-newsrooms-to-better-serve-the-disability-community/). A digital tool kit for journalists (but helpful for writers in general).

The Disability Visibility Project (https://disabilityvisibilityproject.com). "An online community dedicated to creating, sharing, and amplifying disability media and culture."

Job Accommodation Network (https://askjan.org). Resources on obtaining workplace accommodations.

National Parks Interagency Access Pass (https://nps.gov/subjects/accessibility/interagency-access-pass.htm). Free passes to the national parks are available for US citizens or permanent residents with permanent disabilities.

The Neurodiversity Alliance (https://thendalliance.org/). A nonprofit organization whose mission is to "improve the educational experience and outcomes of students who learn differently, while growing the neurodiversity movement for a more equitable and inclusive society for all."

Understood (https://www.understood.org/). A nonprofit organization "empowering the 70 million people with learning and thinking differences in the United States. We provide free, expert-vetted resources and support so people who learn and think differently can thrive—in school, at work, and throughout life."

Directories

Directory of Occupational Therapists (https://otpotential.com/occupational-therapy-directory)

Directory of Therapists and Coaches at CHADD (https://chadd.org/professional-directory)

Professional Association of ADHD Coaches (http://www.paaccoaches.org/)

Professional Directory at ADDA (https://add.org/professional-directory)

Coworking/Body Doubling Spaces

Virtual

Caveday (https://www.caveday.org/)

Flow Club (https://www.flow.club/)

FLOWN (https://flown.com)

Focusmate (https://www.focusmate.com/)

Physical

Coworker (https://www.coworker.com/)
Spaces (https://www.spacesworks.com/)
WeWork (https://www.wework.com/)

Literary Spaces for ND Writing

ANMLY (https://anmly.org/). An online magazine "committed to actively seeking out and promoting the work of marginalized and underrepresented artists, including especially people of color, women, queer, disabled, neurodivergent, and gender nonconforming artists."

Milkweed Editions' Multiverse Series (https://milkweed.org/multiverse). "A literary series devoted to different ways of languaging. . . . Multiverse primarily emerges from the practices and creativity of neurodivergent, autistic, neuroqueer, mad, nonspeaking, and disabled cultures."

Unrestricted Interest (https://www.unrestrictedinterest.com/). An organization "devoted to neurodivergent listening, learning, and languaging" through a micropress, online publications, a Substack, and events.

Wild-Wired: Neurodivergent and Neuroqueer Poetics (https://medium.com/anomalyblog/wild-wired-neurodivergent-and-neuroqueer-poetics-73cb42640f0d). A column that "seeks submissions of poems and poetic prose from neurodivergent writers."

Wordgathering: A Journal of Disability Poetry and Literature (https://wordgathering.com/). "A digital, Open Access, biannual journal of disability poetry, literature, and the arts."

Zoeglossia (https://www.zoeglossia.org/). "A literary organization that is seeking to pioneer an inclusive space for poets with disabilities." Publishes poems online and holds an annual retreat.

Apps, Digital Tools, and Gadgets

Bullet Journal (https://bulletjournal.com/). A handwritten style of planning that many ADHDers love. For less elaborate versions, search online for "simplified or minimal bullet journal techniques" (such as https://www.thelazygeniuscollective.com/blog/how-to-bullet-journal).

Cube Timer (https://mooastime.shop/shop/mooas-timer/). A simple cube timer from Mooas with preset time options; just flip the cube to start and stop.

Goblin.Tools (https://www.goblin.tools/). "A collection of small, simple, single-task tools, mostly designed to help neurodivergent people with tasks they find overwhelming or difficult." Free online or available as an inexpensive app.

InFlow (https://www.getinflow.io/). An ADHD coaching app. Free to download but requires a subscription to use.

Otter AI (https://otter.ai/). An AI note-taking and transcription program. Free, with a paid subscription option for more capabilities.

Pomofocus (http://www.pomofocus.io/). A Pomodoro-method online timer for tracking twenty-five-minute work sessions followed by five- or fifteen-minute breaks. Free, with a paid premium version.

Time Timer (https://www.timetimer.com/collections/applications). Free app version of the classic visual timer. Physical timers are also available for purchase at this site.

Trello (https://trello.com/). Software and app for managing tasks and projects on your own or with others. Free, with subscriptions for more capabilities.

An ADHD Glossary

ableism. The belief, conscious or unconscious, that there is one standard or superior type of body or mind and that systems should be designed to meet the needs of those who fit the perceived norm. **Internalized ableism** refers to how this belief can cause those with cognitive or physical disabilities to view themselves negatively and work to mask their differences rather than critiquing ableist systems. **Anti-ableism** is the belief that all bodies and minds have inherent value and that systems should be designed so all can navigate them with ease and be allowed to flourish.

accommodations. Adjustments aimed at making existing systems (such as schools or workplaces) easier for disabled individuals to navigate. Accommodations can never fully close the gap since the systems that necessitate them were typically designed around ableist principles, but they can help. The four main types of accommodations are **presentation** (adjusting how information is presented), **response** (adjusting how an individual is expected to demonstrate their knowledge of a topic), **setting** (adjustments to one's environment), and **timing and scheduling** (adjusting expectations around time and schedules).

ADHD. Attention-deficit/hyperactivity disorder is the medical term for a neurotype characterized by attention variability and/or hyperactivity-impulsivity severe enough to impact everyday functioning, such as in school, at work, or in social situations. ADHD is diagnosed in three subtypes: **inattentive type**, which is a misnomer—in fact, this type appears as a variability or excess of attention rather than a lack; **hyperactive-impulsive type**, which is marked by a variability or abundance of motor or verbal activity, spontaneous decision-making, and instinctive response; and **combined type**, in which characteristics of both the above types are found. In the past, separate terms and diagnoses were used to distinguish between types with hyperactivity (ADHD) and without (ADD), but the term ADHD is currently used to include all subtypes.

ADHD hacks. Strategies employed by individuals to bring their physical and virtual spaces into better alignment with the way their brain works in order to enhance comfort and improve workflow.

ADHD tax. Unplanned expenditures of time, money, and energy that are the result of bumping up against a world that is not designed for those with ADHD.

AuDHD. A portmanteau that describes individuals who are on the autism spectrum and have ADHD.

body doubling. Having another person in your presence—in person or virtually—as you complete a task in order to increase your motivation and productivity.

bullet journaling. A flexible method designed by someone with ADHD for recording and organizing tasks, ideas, schedules, and doodles in one place.

coaching and **cognitive behavioral therapy (CBT)**. The two most common forms of therapeutic intervention for people with ADHD. Both ADHD coaches and CBT therapists can help individuals with ADHD develop skills, change negative thought patterns, and accomplish personal and professional goals.

co-occurring conditions. ADHD often appears with a range of other co-occurring or comorbid conditions, most notably anxiety, depression, and being on the autism spectrum. Other co-occurring conditions include **rejection sensitivity dysphoria (RSD)**, a heightened emotional response to real or perceived rejection; **oppositional defiance disorder (ODD)**, characterized by acting out or clashing with authority; **obsessive-compulsive disorder (OCD)** and compulsive body-focused repetitive behaviors such as **trichotillomania** and **dermatillomania**; learning disorders such as **dyslexia** and **dyscalculia**; and hormone-related mood disorders such as **premenstrual dysphoric disorder (PMDD)**, **postpartum depression (PPD)**, and increased severity of ADHD symptoms during perimenopause and menopause.

deficit framing. Viewing differences as limitations rather than unique attributes. **Strength/asset framing**, on the other hand, focuses on the strengths and skills people bring to any situation.

disability. A physical or mental impairment that substantially limits one or more major life activities. ADHD is a recognized disability in the United States under the Americans with Disabilities Act (ADA) and the Rehabilitation Act of 1973.

disability justice. Unlike disability rights, which is based on a single identity, disability justice is a movement that is centered around recognizing that we have multiple overlapping identities, each of which can be a site of privilege or oppression, and that those who are most impacted by ableism and systemic oppression—including sick and disabled queer, trans, Black, and brown people—should be at the forefront in decision-making that disproportionately affects them.

dopamine. A neurotransmitter that is responsible for feelings of pleasure and reward. Research shows that people with ADHD have a dopamine deficiency.

executive dysfunction. Difficulty with the cognitive processes required to organize thoughts and activities, prioritize tasks, manage time efficiently, and make decisions.

hyperfocus. Highly focused attention that lasts for an extended period. During a period of hyperfocus, one may lose track of time, forget obligations, and be unaware of one's physical environment and bodily needs. Hyperfocus also allows people with ADHD to sometimes accomplish an unusual amount of work in a short time.

hypervigilance. An extreme awareness of your surroundings, people, and/or hidden dangers; a constant self-surveillance undertaken by many individuals with ADHD in order to correct and conceal errors and vulnerabilities.

intersectionality. A term coined in 1989 by Professor Kimberlé Crenshaw that refers to the ways that race, class, gender, and other characteristics/categories/conditions "intersect" with one another, impacting people in ways that attention to any one category often erases.

masking. Any behavior that a neurodivergent person uses to conceal thoughts, emotions, and behaviors that might not conform to societal expectations.

medication. ADHD medications fall into two categories: stimulant and non-stimulant. In both cases, they increase neurotransmitter chemicals in the brain, which can help with focus, impulse control, and executive function. Studies have shown medication to be helpful for a high percentage of people with ADHD. Some people with ADHD find medications to be extremely beneficial and liken them to wearing glasses to correct vision, while others prefer to avoid medication and may use alternatives such as cognitive behavior therapy (CBT), ADHD coaching, and ADHD-friendly accommodations.

neurodiversity. This term, coined by sociologist Judy Singer in 1997, reframes neurological difference as a kind of natural variety rather than as a disorder or impairment. Many people with ADHD or other cognitive differences refer to themselves as **neurodivergent/neurodiverse (ND)** or as having a specific

neurotype. Those with more common and socially accepted cognitive patterns might in turn be referred to as **neurotypical** (**NT**). An expectation that everyone's cognition works the same way can be referred to as **neuronormativity**.

neurospicy. A playful and positive self-referential slang term for neurodivergent people, often expressed online with the chili pepper emoji.

regulation of emotions (also **dysregulation**, **self-regulation**). The ability to manage and respond to emotional situations. **Dysregulation** refers to a state of intense or uncontrolled emotion, or an inability to control emotional responses. **Self-regulation** is a skill one can develop to manage and modulate one's own emotional responses.

sensory overload. Overwhelm and exhaustion resulting from taking in more sensory data than the brain is able to process.

shame spiral. Intense feelings of shame, guilt, or humiliation, which may make a person with ADHD avoid the related situation entirely rather than address it.

spoon theory. A term coined by American writer Christine Miserandino in 2003. According to this theory, a person starts each day with a fixed number of **spoons**, representing physical and mental energy. This metaphor illustrates how disabilities and challenges of many kinds can limit the number of spoons one has to begin with and can accelerate the depletion of those resources. "All out of spoons" has become a way to describe a total depletion of energy due to managing extra, often invisible challenges in everyday life.

stimming. Repetitive behaviors that are self-soothing and self-stimulating. People with ADHD may "stim" to release energy or to stay focused. For example, knitting, doodling, or using a fidget toy may help individuals with ADHD listen to a lecture or sit still in a meeting; jiggling a knee or humming might appear as a more involuntary type of stimming.

success amnesia. The inability to remember one's own accomplishments and successes (also called **accomplishment amnesia**).

task paralysis. An inability to start or finish a task due to information overload, executive dysfunction, and/or anxiety. Also called **ADHD paralysis, decision paralysis**.

thought patterns. The characteristics that come with ADHD can affect cognition in many ways. Troublesome thought patterns may include **racing thoughts**

(a constant stream of thoughts often related to worry or catastrophizing); **rumination** (excessive worry or overthinking about a single thing); and **intrusive thoughts** (uninvited thoughts that can be disturbing and tough to get rid of). More beneficial thought patterns that are enhanced in ADHD include **cognitive flexibility** (thinking "outside the box," or beyond conventional approaches); **cognitive persistence** (working at a problem until a solution is found); **associative thinking** (jumping from one idea to another and making unexpected connections); **pattern recognition** (noticing patterns and connections that most people might miss); and **conceptual expansion** (being able to think beyond existing paradigms).

time agnosia. The inability to correctly perceive the passage of time or to accurately estimate how much time is needed for a given task. Although the term "time blindness" has often been used to describe this concept, disability advocacy groups recognize it as an ableist term.

twice-exceptional. A term for people who are intellectually gifted and also have a learning disability or neuro-difference. The unusual abilities of twice-exceptional (or **2e**) people are often obscured by the challenges their co-occurring conditions present at work or in school. Giftedness can also obscure symptoms of ADHD, making it hard to identify and diagnose.

working memory. The mechanism by which we are able to hold multiple pieces of information, then organize and use that information. People with ADHD may struggle with working memory, which is a key component of executive function.

Contributors

Robin Black's story collection, *If I Loved You, I Would Tell You This*, was a finalist for the Frank O'Connor International Short Story Award. Her novel, *Life Drawing*, was long-listed for multiple awards and named a Best Book of the Year by NPR, among others. An essay collection, *Crash Course: Essays from Where Writing and Life Collide*, came out in 2016, followed by the harder to categorize conversation with a book, *Virginia Woolf's Mrs. Dalloway, Bookmarked*, in 2022. Robin, who has taught most recently in the Rutgers Camden MFA Program for Writers, lives in Philadelphia with her husband and is at work on a novel.

lawrence-minh bùi davis is a refugee diaspore, curator, editor, writer, troublemaker, and cinnamon roll who lives as a guest on the ancestral lands of the Piscataway Nation, sometimes also known as Prince George's County, Maryland, a place nestled in the shadows of various colonial enterprises. A cofounder of the arts anti-profit AALR (2009), the Asian American Literature Festival (2017), the Center for Refugee Poetics (2018), and the Asian American Lit Fest Collective (2023), he believes in stewardship of literature as social and ethical ecosystem and growing collective responsibility for what we read and write, and why. Sometimes you can see new things by the light of his ADHD.

Teresa Dzieglewicz is a poet, educator, and lover of rivers and prairies. She is a fellow with Black Earth Institute, a Poet-in-Residence at the Chicago Poetry Center, and part of the founding team of Mní Wičhóni Nakíčižiŋ Wóuŋspe (Defenders of the Water School). Her first book of poetry, *Something Small of How to See a River*, was selected by Tyehimba Jess for the Dorset Prize (Tupelo Press). Her first children's book, cowritten with Kimimila Locke, is forthcoming from Chronicle Books. She has won a Pushcart Prize, Best New Poets, the Ginkgo Prize, the Auburn Witness Poetry Prize, and the Palette Poetry Prize, and she has received fellowships from the Elizabeth George Foundation, the Community of Writers at Tahoe, the Kimmel Harding Nelson Center for the Arts, and Brooklyn Poets.

Elizabeth Ito has been working as a creator, writer, director, and storyboard artist in the animation industry since 2004. She's worked on TV, feature, and commercial projects. Elizabeth is the creator of the award-winning short *Welcome to My Life*, the second-most viewed short in Cartoon Network history. She also received an Emmy for her directing work on *Adventure Time*. Her first series, *City of Ghosts* for Netflix, premiered in 2021 and won a Peabody Award and two Emmys (for directing and best animated children's show) in 2022. She also directed a music video for The Linda Lindas. Currently, she is living in Los Angeles, working from home, and trying to stay hydrated.

Douglas Kearney has published books ranging from poetry to essays. His newest, *I Imagine I Been Science Fiction Always*, is a collection of visual poetry. In 2023 *Optic Subwoof* won the Poetry Foundation's Pegasus Award for Poetry Criticism and the CLMP Firecracker Award for Creative Nonfiction. His seventh book, *Sho*, is a Griffin Poetry Prize and Minnesota Book Award winner. Kearney has been awarded the Whiting Writers Award and the Cy Twombly Award for Poetry from the Foundation for Contemporary Arts. His residencies/fellowships include Cave Canem Foundation, the Robert Rauschenberg Foundation, and the McKnight Foundation. He is a Samuel Russell Chair in the Humanities in the College of Liberal Arts and Professor of English at the University of Minnesota Twin Cities.

David Kessler MA, LPC, is a practicing therapist with over a decade of clinical experience; an ADHD and trauma expert; and a nationally recognized speaker and ADHD advocate. He cohosts the ADHD podcast *Something Shiny* and lives with his partner Robin in Chicago.

Jennifer L. Knox is the author of five poetry collections, most recently *Crushing It* (Copper Canyon Press, 2020). Her poems have appeared four times in The Best American Poetry series and in anthologies such as *You Are Here: Poetry in the Natural World*, *The 2022 Pushcart Prize: Best of the Small Presses*, and *Great American Prose Poems: From Poe to Present*. Her work has also been featured in *The New York Times*, *The New Yorker*, *Orion*, *American Poetry Review*, *McSweeney's*, and *BOMB*. She lives in central Iowa, where she wrangles spice blends in a very tiny pen at Saltlickers.

Jami Nakamura Lin is the author of the illustrated speculative memoir *The Night Parade*, the winner of the 2024 Chicago Review of Books Award for Nonfiction. *The Night Parade* was named a Best Book of 2023 by *The Boston Globe* and a Best Memoir by *Vulture/New York Magazine*, and received starred reviews from *Kirkus*, *Publishers Weekly*, and *Library Journal*. Jami has received support from organizations including the National Endowment for the Arts/Japan-US Friendship Commission, the Folger Shakespeare Library, MacDowell, Yaddo, Sewanee, We Need

Diverse Books, and the Illinois Arts Council. Her essays and stories have been published in *The New York Times*, *Sewanee Review*, and *Passages North*, among others. She teaches at StoryStudio Chicago and is working on her next book.

Rebecca Makkai is the author of *The New York Times*' best-selling *I Have Some Questions for You* as well as four other works of fiction. Her last novel, *The Great Believers*, one of *The New York Times*' Best Books of the 21st Century, was a finalist for both the 2019 Pulitzer Prize and the 2018 National Book Award, and was the winner of the ALA Andrew Carnegie Medal for Excellence in Fiction and the *Los Angeles Times* Book Prize in Fiction, among other honors. A 2022 Guggenheim Fellow, Rebecca teaches graduate fiction writing at Middlebury College, Northwestern University, and the Bennington Writing Seminars, and she is Artistic Director of StoryStudio Chicago.

Kwoya Fagin Maples is a poet, woodworker, and teacher of creative writing. She is the author of *Long Eye*, forthcoming from Hub City Press in 2026, and coeditor of *I Witness: An Anthology of Documentary Poetry*, forthcoming from Wesleyan University Press. Her debut collection, *Mend* (University Press of Kentucky, 2018), was a finalist for the 2019 Hurston/Wright Legacy Award for Poetry. She teaches in the MFA program for Creative Writing at the University of Alabama.

Rainie Oet writes fiction and poetry for adults and young readers. She is the author of the middle grade novel-in-verse *Glitch Girl!* (Kokila), the picture books *Robin's Worlds* and *Monster Seek* (Astra), and three books of poetry: *Glorious Veils of Diane* (Carnegie Mellon), *Inside Ball Lightning* (SEMO), and *Porcupine in Freefall* (Bright Hill Book Prize). Her work also appears in *Strange Horizons*; *The Poetry Review*; *Puerto Del Sol* (2019 Poetry Contest); *He, She, They, Us: Queer Poems* (Macmillan); and *You're Never Too Much: Poems for Every Emotion* (Macmillan), among other publications. She received her MFA at Syracuse University, where she was awarded the Shirley Jackson Prize in Fiction. Read more at rainieoet.com.

Khadijah Queen holds a PhD in English from the University of Denver. She is the author of seven books of poetry and prose, including *I'm So Fine: A List of Famous Men & What I Had On* (YesYes Books, 2017), praised in *O Magazine*, *The New Yorker, Rain Taxi*, and elsewhere as "quietly devastating" and "a portrait of defiance that turns the male gaze inside out." In 2025 the Foundation for Contemporary Arts recognized Queen's work with the Cy Twombly Award in Poetry. Her memoir, *Between the Devil and the Deep Blue Sea*, about her time in the US Navy alongside short histories of women sailors, was published by Legacy Lit/Hachette in 2025.

Emily Stoddard is a writer and artist in northern Michigan. She is the author of *Surfacing*, a book of closing practices for creative writers, and *Divination with a*

Human Heart Attached, a poetry book. She is a past recipient of the Developmental Editing Fellowship for Emerging Writers in creative nonfiction from the *Kenyon Review*, and her work appears in *Belt Magazine*, *The Baltimore Review*, *Radar*, *Whitefish Review*, and elsewhere. Read more at emilystoddard.com.

Doug Van Gundy directs the low-residency MFA program in creative writing at West Virginia Wesleyan College. His poems and essays have appeared in many journals, including *The Oxford American*, *The Guardian*, *Poetry*, *Poets & Writers*, and *Ecotone*. His first book of poems, *A Life Above Water*, was published by Red Hen Press. He is the coeditor of *Eyes Glowing at the Edge of the Woods: Contemporary Writing from West Virginia*, published by Vandalia Press. In addition to writing and teaching, Doug is an award-winning old-time musician whose music has been featured on three CDs, several films, and National Public Radio's Mountain Stage. He plays fiddle, guitar, and mandolin in the duo Born Old.

About the Editors

Lisa Van Orman Hadley is the author of *Irreversible Things* (Howling Bird Press, 2019), a novel-in-stories that weaves together memoir, fiction, and the fiction of remembering. *Irreversible Things* was awarded the Howling Bird Press Fiction Prize, the AML Special Award in Literature, two Midwest Book Awards silver medals, the Larry Levis Post-Graduate Stipend, and a Barbara Deming Memorial Fund grant. Her stories have appeared in the *New England Review*, the *Collagist*, and *Epoch* and have been shortlisted in *Ploughshares* and *Glimmer Train*. She works as a freelance editor and is currently writing a memoir about growing up with undiagnosed ADHD. She lives in the foothills of Salt Lake City with her husband, cat, and thirteen-year-old twins. Her special interests include rock climbing, knitting, and cramming as many plants into her house as possible.

Chloe Martinez is a poet, translator, and scholar of South Asian religions. She is the author of two books of poetry, *Ten Thousand Selves* (The Word Works, 2021) and *Corner Shrine* (Backbone Press, 2020), and the translator of *Songs of Mirabai* (New Directions, 2026). Her work has appeared in *Ploughshares*, *Poetry*, *The Common*, *Agni*, *Sierra Magazine*, and elsewhere, and has been featured on Poetry Daily and *The Slowdown* podcast. She serves as assistant editor for *Beloit Poetry Journal* and poetry editor for the *Journal of Feminist Studies in Religion*, and is associate director of programming for the Center for Writing and Public Discourse at Claremont McKenna College. She lives with her husband and two daughters in Claremont, California, on the traditional lands of the Tongva/Gabrielino people.